Counselling People with Cancer

Counselling People with Cancer

Mary Burton
Chartered Clinical Psychologist and Psychotherapist in Private Practice
London, UK

and

Maggie Watson
Consultant Clinical Psychologist
The Royal Marsden NHS Trust and Institute of Cancer Research
Sutton, UK

JOHN WILEY & SONS
Chichester • New York • Weinheim • Brisbane • Singapore • Toronto

Copyright 1988 by John Wiley & Sons Ltd,
     Baffins Lane, Chichester,
     West Sussex PO19 1UD, England

     National 01243 779777
     International (+44) 1243 779777
     e-mail (for orders and customer service enquiries):
     cs-books@wiley.co.uk
     Visit our Home Page on http://www.wiley.co.uk
        or http://www.wiley.com

Other Wiley Editorial Offices

John Wiley & Sons, Inc., 605 Third Avenue,
New York, NY 10158-0012, USA

WILEY-VCH Verlag GmbH, Pappelallee 3,
D-69469 Weinheim, Germany

Jacaranda Wiley Ltd, 33 Park Road, Milton,
Queensland 4064, Australia

John Wiley & Sons (Asia) Pte Ltd, 2 Clementi Loop #02-01,
Jin Xing Distripark, Singapore 129 809

John Wiley & Sons (Canada) Ltd, 22 Worcester Road,
Rexdale, Ontario M9W 1L1, Canada

Library of Congress Cataloging-in-Publication Data

Burton, Mary, clinical psychologist.
 Counselling people with cancer/Mary Burton, Maggie Watson.
  p. cm.
 Includes bibliographical references and index.
 ISBN 0-471-97813-2 (pbk : alk. paper)
 1. Cancer–Patients–Counseling of. I. Watson, M. II. Title.
 [DNLM: 1. Neoplasms–psychology. 2. Counseling–methods.
 3. Psychotherapy–methods. QZ 200 B974c 1998]
 RC262.B87 1998
 616.99'4'0019–dc21
 DNLM/DLC
 for Library of Congress   97–34810
                       CIP

British Library Cataloguing in Publication Data

A catalogue record for this book is available from the British Library

ISBN 0 471 97813 2

Typeset in 11/13pt Palatino from the authors' disks by Acorn Bookwork, Salisbury, Wilts

Contents

Foreword ix

Preface xiii

Acknowledgements xv

1 **Having Cancer: The Patient's Experience** **1**
Perceptions of cancer as a disease 1
The experience of becoming ill 4
The experience of having cancer 7

2 **Cancer Treatments and Psychological Problems** **14**
Disease stage 14
Cancer treatments 15
The treatment process 16
Psychological aspects of cancer surgery 18
Effects of radiotherapy and chemotherapy 23
Bone marrow transplant and hormonal therapies 24
Psychological problems 26
Suicide risk 28
Patients at risk of psychological problems 28
Common themes to patients' problems 29

3 **Coping with Cancer** **34**
Styles of coping 34
Denial as a response to cancer 36
What is denial? 36
Dealing with denial and avoidance 38
Dealing with anger 40

4 Family Issues   **43**
Cancer is a family problem   43
Family members' reactions to a loved one's
  cancer   44
Difference in coping style between patients and
  their partners   46
The conspiracy of silence   47
Families at risk   48
Children's reactions to a parent's cancer   50
Cultural variations in family response   52
Staff relationships with family members   53

5 Couples' Issues and Psychosexual Problems   **55**
The impact of cancer on the couple   55
Psychosexual issues in cancer   56
Psychosexual aspects of colostomy   62
Psychosexual aspects of mastectomy   66

6 Communication Problems   **69**
Disclosing the diagnosis and prognosis   69
Breaking bad news   75
How emotions limit communication and
  understanding   78
'Am I dying, doctor?'   85
Specific communication problems   86
Guidelines for information-giving   89
Informed consent   91
Discussing therapeutic options: giving patients
  choice   91

7 Counselling over the Course of the Illness   **94**
The onset of cancer in context   94
Cancer recurrence   96
Spiritual needs of cancer patients   97
The dying patient   99
Communication with dying patients   102
The dying patient's family   105
Psychological adaptation to death   109
Bereavement   111

8   **The Psychodynamic Model**   113
    The psychodynamic life narrative   113
    Brief focused psychodynamic psychotherapy   117
    The psychodynamic formulation   123

9   **The Client-centred Model**   126
    Establishing a counselling relationship: general
        principles   126
    The first counselling session   131
    Helpers' resistances to listening to feelings   134
    Patients who do not want counselling   136
    Talking with people about their feelings: a practical
        guide   137

10 **The Cognitive–Behavioural Model**   150
    Ventilation of emotions   151
    Behavioural techniques   152
    Spouse or partner as co-therapist   154
    Cognitive techniques   155

11 **Group Therapy**   160
    What type of group?   160
    Running a support group   162

12 **Professional Issues**   171
    Setting up a service   171
    Service evaluation   172
    Measures of psychological morbidity   173
    Economic measures   174
    Supervision   174
    Confidentiality   175
    The counselling contract   176

References   178

Index   195

Foreword

It has been a great pleasure for me to see the development of psychosocial oncology on a global scale over the past twenty years. Based in large part on the reports from increasingly sophisticated research studies in the field, and from the growing numbers of oncology centres which have psychosocial units, the patient's psychological state and level of distress have today become a legitimate part of the treating team's total medical care. The psychological dimension has become a sub-speciality of oncology with its own body of research and field of scientific inquiry. Quality of life is an important outcome variable in the clinical trials which determine the new standard treatment for specific types and stages of cancer. It helps to guide treatment decisions for patients who face new treatments with a range of side effects. The epidemiological studies of the nature and prevalence of distress in patients, by site, stage and treatment of disease, have largely informed psychologists and oncologists about the common psychological problems and psychiatric disorders. We know more about what coping style and which resources lead to a better psychological state and increased quality of life. These first steps of defining the clinical psychological issues have rapidly been followed by many studies of the different types of psychosocial intervention designed to reduce distress and enhance coping and adaptation to illness.

There is no better time for this thoughtful volume on counselling to appear. Written by two of the world's outstanding psychosocial oncologists, Mary Burton and Maggie Watson bring a wealth of clinical and research experience to this important topic. They have both written widely about counselling, and have helped to develop counselling methods for patients with cancer. This volume is a treasure for the clinician who wishes to learn as much as possible about the underpinnings and application of types of psychotherapy and counselling, while also being informed about the range of issues that arise daily in clinical counselling with patients. The authors carefully outline the emotional experience, the families' responses, the pitfalls of poor communication and the particularly critical component of the doctor-patient interaction – as well as the positive benefits which result from a respectful and trusting relationship characterized by open dialogue. The special issues faced by couples in which one partner has cancer are reviewed, with particular emphasis on the psychosexual issues that are often overlooked because patients are embarrassed to bring up the topic and doctors too often don't ask. Guidelines for the counselling of patients at different stages of illness receive appropriate attention – the newly diagnosed patient faces different issues and needs different counselling compared to the patient with advanced disease.

The heart of the book, which psychosocial oncologists will find extremely valuable, is the discussion of the models of individual counselling: the psychodynamic, client-centred, and cognitive-behavioural models are all covered, as are the issues associated with group therapy which is so widely used today. Professional aspects of the psychosocial oncologist's role also receive attention: how do you set up a service, manage it and run it in the most confidential, economic and prudent way? These aspects of counselling have, to date, received little attention. The newly qualified clinician must have this book to be fully prepared for the psychological care of patients with cancer. The overview will equip him or her with the knowledge and skills needed to give good psychosocial care. This volume should become required reading in the model curriculum for those training in psychosocial oncology. Experienced clinicians will find the insights of these two seasoned psychosocial oncologists refreshing; they will find a thoroughly readable, useful review of the psychosocial domain and the counselling models available today. Clinicians in oncology whose backgrounds lie in oncology, nursing or social work will find the book free of technical jargon and a useful guide to the psychological side of patient care.

The field of psychosocial oncology has been enriched by this landmark volume. It is the first book of its kind to provide an in-depth analysis of current counselling models, and offers a crisp critique of them along with recommendations for their use, based on the authors' knowledge of the theoretical issues and their clinical experience. As one of the pioneers in psychosocial oncology, I am pleased to see that the future of the field is secure. Burton and Watson have shown that counselling has come of age and can be counted among the range of therapies from which patients with cancer will benefit.

Jimmie C. Holland, MD
Chairman, Department of Psychiatry & Behavioral Sciences
Memorial Sloan-Kettering Cancer Center
New York

Preface

This book is not aimed at any specific professional group. Anyone who asks themselves, 'How can I help with the emotional and humane side of dealing with cancer?' should find the issues described here of interest:

- how to explore the problems facing cancer patients and their families

- how best to address patients' psychological needs

- how the skills of counselling can be specifically adapted to meet the special needs of people who have cancer.

The book emphasizes the three mainstream models of individual counselling: client- or person-centred (humanistic), psychodynamic and cognitive–behavioural models. Some attention is also given to working with groups, families and couples and to the treatment of psychosexual problems. Basic communication skills are included as well as formal counselling techniques.

Books describing clinical practice are helpful because they provide guidelines and a framework or describe techniques along with the difficulties that might be encountered. They can provide a springboard from which to launch into the practical work, and a reference source. There is no substitute for the direct experience of working with people who have cancer and developing skills on a trial and error basis. This book is no exception in being an adjunct to practical skills training, but it also offers suggestions for the supervision of counselling work and further development of psychological and counselling skills.

Framework of the Book

Chapter 1 begins with the patient's experience of having cancer, including lay perceptions of the illness. Chapter 2 describes the three principal cancer treatments (surgery, radiotherapy and chemotherapy) and related psychological problems, including common themes. Chapter 3 focuses on the coping styles of people with cancer as a basis for understanding how these influence behaviour and emotional responses. Chapter 4 describes the impact of cancer on the family and Chapter 5 focuses on couples' issues and psychosexual problems. Chapter 6 is devoted to communication problems with cancer patients, including information giving, the bad news interview, informed consent and patient involvement in the choice of treatment.

Counselling over the course of the illness is described in Chapter 7, including a discussion of the spiritual needs of cancer patients and dying patients and their families. Chapter 8 describes brief psychodynamic models of counselling, and Chapter 9 presents the client-centred reflection-of-feelings model. Chapter 10 provides a rationale for a more directive and structured approach based on cognitive–behavioural methods. Chapter 11 describes group therapy models, and the final chapter deals with professional issues and service development.

All case histories cited have been changed to protect the identity of the patients and their families and in some instances they represent a compilation of different patients' cases.

Acknowledgements

We are grateful to the inspiration of Dr. Steven Greer and the late Professor Tim McElwain who considered that psychological care for patients was of importance. More than anything, the unsung heroes and heroines of this book are the patients and their families who have shared with us their experiences and feelings over the years.

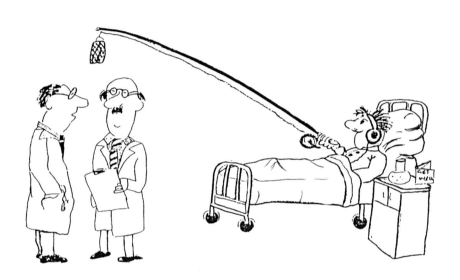

Reproduced by kind permission of Basildon Hospital. Source unknown.

1
Having Cancer: The Patient's Experience

Perceptions of Cancer as a Disease

Cancer is a common disease. One in five of the population in Europe, the USA and the developed countries will die from it (Cancer Research Campaign 1989) and one in three of the population will develop it in their lifetime. Although often perceived as one disease, it is a number of diseases subsumed within one diagnostic label. It is often considered more frightening than other equally lethal illnesses. As one patient put it, 'Cancer is everyone's worst nightmare'. There is a mythology surrounding cancer, with many superstitious beliefs. This arises to some extent because it is poorly understood. Cancer is associated with prolonged suffering, with wasting away, and with a slow lingering death. Understanding disease mechanisms can demystify illness. While cancer remains poorly understood, superstitious beliefs are likely to continue.

Much has been written about why cancer is such a fearful disease. This may be because it seems to ravage silently from within. It is an unseen enemy; it is part of our body, yet not part of our body. We use powerful combative language to describe it. We talk about cancer 'victims', about 'fighting' cancer and about how cancer 'invades' the body. We are none of us wholly immune to the fears. Perhaps more than anything else, fear arises from the perception that cancer may be uncontrollable and the feeling that little can be done to stay its course. Cancer is sometimes seen as medicine's failure.

Cancer, as a disease that predominates among the elderly, is likely to continue to be a major cause of death in western populations. It has been suggested that as the number of elderly people increases so too will the prevalence rates of many common cancers. There seems no reason to believe that its prevalence will decrease over the next 50 years or so. The need to accept that it will not be possible in the forseeable future to cure all cancers is an important reason to support a more holistic model of patient care that encompasses psychological support and a need to use medicine to help to improve the quality of life. This view has recently received some support from the UK Government's Medical Officer: the Calman Report (Department of Health 1995) on cancer services draws attention to the importance of taking account of the psychological needs of patients at all points in their cancer career. With this more broad-ranging approach comes the need to develop counselling and communication skills in those professional groups having regular contact with people who have cancer.

There is a need in 'high-tech' medicine to rediscover what Jewson (1976) has called 'bedside medicine', the idea that psyche and soma are intimately inter-related. Although it may seem that the person has been replaced by the cell as the fundamental unit of life in medicine, it is important to remain in touch with the needs of the patient as a person and to try to practice the most humane form of medicine.

Given the strong emotions that the disease can evoke, it is not surprising to learn that the level of psychological morbidity among cancer patients and their families is high. One frequently quoted study of newly diagnosed patients placed the prevalence rate for adjustment disorders (the predominant psychiatric diagnosis reported) at 46% (Derogatis *et al.* 1983) and more recent evidence confirms the high rates of distress (Parle *et al.* 1994). However, serious disturbance is more often confined to between 10 and 15% of patients (Dean 1987; Watson *et al.* 1991). Given the large numbers of people diagnosed with cancer, this represents a very substantial mental health problem. These prevalence rates for psychological morbidity vary according to the type of cancer and the stage of the disease, being somewhat higher in people with more advanced disease.

There is, of course, a brighter side to this gloomy picture. There are people who make a full recovery and are considered cured, and those who, although not formally considered to be 'cured', nevertheless live for many years with their disease and maintain a good quality of life. For these patients, rehabilitation is an important goal. However, where the disease is far advanced and life expectancy is short, an important aim is to assist people with cancer to live their lives as fully as possible within the physical constaints of the disease and its treatment.

While many people with cancer cope remarkably well, a substantial minority find it extremely difficult. Counselling and effective psychological care can be of immense benefit and should be considered an integral part of health care. There is a view (Bellet and Maloney 1991) that effective communication will help to prevent some of the documented psychological morbidity and in particular help to reduce anxiety. It is important to try to improve communication skills within those professions dealing with cancer patients and their families. More important, however, is the need to acknowledge that care of the cancer patient must be wide-ranging and should include close attention to the psychological needs of the patient.

Osler (1910) drew attention to the need to understand the psychological dimensions as well as the purely biological aspects of medical care. To develop good communication and counselling skills within the caring professions serves patients well in a range of ways. For doctors, there are strong arguments in favour of integrating communication skills training further into continuing medical education. Fletcher (1980) put this well when he said:

> *Doctors whose sole or major concern is with their patients' physical well-being may well deny that they either wish or need to improve their history-taking skills to encompass their patients' personal problems. But, unless they confine themselves to forms of treatment in which the patient himself has no part to play, they need to learn better methods of exposition to ensure success.*

The Experience of Becoming Ill

Let us take a step backward for a moment and consider the experience of becoming ill. The helper's first task is to climb into the patient's shoes for long enough to sense from the inside a bit of what it is like to be this person at this particular moment. This ability to sense the other person's felt world from the inside is called **empathy**. Empathy differs greatly from **sympathy**, which is closer to pity, feeling sorry for the other or saying, 'Poor you'. Sympathy rarely helps and is often resented, but empathy can make an enormous difference to a person's feeling of well-being, hope and self-esteem. Part of becoming an empathic listener is learning about the experience of illness from the inside. There are a number of well-described changes in us when we fall ill, and an understanding of these will greatly assist us in responding to the cancer patient's needs.

Health care staff working in a hospital setting can easily forget what a strange environment the hospital is to a newly admitted patient.

> *The smells and colours are not the same as at home, the meals are at different times, there are new people to get used to, the world must be viewed from a bed and the horizontal position rather than the vertical one they are used to when they are well, and so on. Furthermore, whereas previously the patients belonged to themselves and took care of their own bodily needs and functions, they are now properties to be cared for, fed, washed, and cleaned. Their privacy is invaded and they must perform the most intimate functions in the presence of others; even that most personal of all things, suffering, has to be gone through in a crowd (Gillis 1972).*
>
> *The world around the person shrinks to a small space, scarcely larger than his own body – the box of tissues on the bed, the bed itself, and perhaps the room ... In health we know we are alive by our connectedness to the world ... In illness, however slight, some of these contacts are lost ... As illness deepens, connections are increasingly cut ... We also lose our sense of omnipotence. Loss of control over the world is another important part of being ill ... The sick represent a threat to the rest of us by making us dangerously aware of the frailty of our own connectedness, the thinness of our shield of omnipotence, the incompetence of reason, and the transience of our control over the world (Cassell 1976).*

When we fall ill, we re-experience emotions of helplessness, passivity and loss that were more appropriate to early childhood. This process is known as **regression**. It is a normal experience in illness and should not be regarded as neurotic. For some helpers, this position of the patient acts as a symbol of their own vulnerability that they wish to deny, impairing their ability to respond to patients at an emotional level. Not wanting to acknowledge their own frailties, they may inappropriately resent the normal process of regression that occurs in illness. They may resent patients' dependency upon them, or respond angrily to patients' demands.

Illness often intensifies pre-existing personality traits. People who tend to be passive or dependent in their relationships may become almost childlike in their helplessness, or they may develop a contentious, care-demanding attitude. Those prone to distrust may become almost paranoid about their care. Those who require a high degree of orderliness may refuse to relinquish management of the illness to the doctor. Some may perceive the illness as a punishment for past misdeeds. Others may equate it with the loss of love from significant people in their lives. All of these reactions can lead to people being seen as 'problem patients' (Corradi 1983). Problem patients actually need more care and attention than non-problem patients but they are often unpopular with staff. Sensitive listeners can be alert to these common reactions to illness and explore them meaningfully with the patient. For example:

> You've always been very independent, and this illness forces you to be dependent on us, which you seem to be finding very difficult.

> You've wanted your family to look after you for a long time, and now you're ill, there is a lot of satisfaction in being looked after.

> There seems to be a feeling that this illness is a punishment for something terrible you did in the past.

> It seems that you are very angry about having this illness, and one way or another you seem to be expressing some of that anger with us, around your treatment.

The acknowledgment of these feelings, as long as they are offered tentatively and supportively, can be of enormous benefit to the patient and can improve patient–staff interaction. Consider the following example: (Dubovsky and Weissberg 1982).

Mrs. R was found to be suffering from acute leukaemia and chemotherapy was instituted. Then, the patient seemed to undergo a personality change. She became irritable and complained constantly. Her ability to tolerate frustration and pain decreased dramatically, and she burst into tears if she experienced nausea after receiving chemotherapy. She rang for the nurses incessantly and never seemed satisfied with the care she received. Although she originally encouraged her husband to go home and look after the children, she now cannot stand to have him out of her sight. Additional history reveals that the patient was the third of seven children of a farming family. She helped to care for the younger children and worked on the farm in addition to going to school. She married at nineteen and one year later had her first child. Her husband describes her as a very independent, unselfish person who hardly ever complains and who is always more interested in others' welfare than her own. He is surprised and frightened by her current behaviour.

It is unhelpful to treat such patients as irascible children, blaming them, admonishing them to control themselves or labelling them psychiatrically. An empathic response to this patient would involve exploring with her the conflicts she is experiencing around assuming the dependent role in hospital as a cancer patient on chemotherapy. Empathic listening along with the setting of appropriate limits and the encouragement of visiting by family and friends will produce a much better result than assuming a critical parental role in such cases.

Among the types of psychological stress to which the hospitalised patient is vulnerable are these: the basic threat to narcissistic integrity; fear of strangers; separation anxiety; fear of the loss of love and approval; fear of the loss of bowel and bladder control, and of the regulation of feeling states; fear of loss of or injury to body parts; reactivation of feelings of guilt and shame; and fears of retaliation for past transgressions (Strain 1978).

All of these anxieties are age-appropriate between birth and 5 years. They may be very difficult indeed for adults to negotiate at 25, 50 or 85. It is beneficial for patients to regress appropriately in the service of their recovery and they may need gentle encouragement to do so. Some cases of noncompliance with treatment are fundamentally about an individual patient's difficulty in assuming the dependency of the patient role and coping with the regression involved in being ill. Careful listening and exploration of the underlying issues can often resolve the non-compliance question. Illness often results in an intensification of a person's characteristic personality style. Different personalities may react differently to illness (Table 1.1) (Geringer and Stern 1986).

An understanding of the range of reactions to illness will help staff to recognize these patterns when they occur and to avoid blaming, judging, avoiding or getting into battles with patients. A tentative reflection-of-feelings response can be very supportive, for example: 'It sounds like one of the worst bits of this illness for you is the loss of control', or 'What seems to be upsetting you most acutely at the moment is how you will feel about your physical attractiveness after this operation'.

Viney, in her book *Images of Illness*, has categorized some of the feelings that arise in people who have fallen ill. These examples of patients' statements may help staff begin to recognize some of the emotional issues facing the cancer patient (Viney 1983).

- Uncertainty: 'It's the type of disease where you won't know how it's going to hit you.'

- Anxiety: 'I'll be scared until this operation is over.'

- Anger: 'I'm fed up with being sick all the time.'

- Helplessness: 'I can't make any long-range plans. I've just stopped living, I guess.'

- Depression: 'I have lost all interest in life. There is no cure for what I've got.'

- Isolation: 'With my problem, you become a social outcast.'

- Humour: 'I've got another wrinkle and that shows I've lived another year.'

The Experience of Having Cancer

'Cancer is the enemy within, a cannibalistic enemy. Cancer is personified' (Cassell 1976). The playwright Dennis Potter in his

Table 1.1   The reaction to illness by different personality types

Personality type	Intrapsychic meaning of illness	Characteristic behaviours during an illness; staff response
Dependent, over-demanding personality	Threat of abandonment	Increased demands, anger and blaming doctors
Compulsive or orderly, controlled personality	Threat of loss of self-control	Increasing rigidity, seeks more information, can be indecisive; illness seen as a loss of control; allow as much control over care as possible
Hysterical or dramatizing personality	Threat to masculinity or femininity	Fear of bodily damage and loss of physical prowess (men); fear of loss of attractiveness (women)
Masochistic or long-suffering, self-sacrificing personality	Deserved punishment for worthlessness, but a permissible way of being cared for	Wish for care often greater than the wish for symptom reduction; patients need to be encouraged to care for themselves
Narcissistic, self-centred personality	Threat to self-image of autonomy or perfection	May alternately idealize and devalue the doctor; illness may intensify the defence of grandiosity: needs to be cared for by 'the best'; may become depressed
Schizoid, aloof personality	Threat of intrusion	Withdraws, denies, asks few questions; requires the maximum privacy, can be reclusive
Paranoid or guarded personality	Threat of attack	Expects the worst in others and then attacks out of proportion to the situation; becomes mistrustful of care-givers, often makes staff angry

last interview called his tumour Rupert (Channel Four Television 1994). To many people, a diagnosis of cancer is tantamount to a death sentence. Many consider it to be a shameful form of 'body rot', something to be hidden away and kept from view, the sinister crab eating away at the body from within. Some will even say, 'We've been a clean-living family. No one in our family has ever had cancer'.

Senescu (1963) described six common responses to the disease:

- the *dependency response*: some patients fight dependency; others almost seem to bask in it

- the feeling of *damage and reduction of self-esteem*: 'I've felt like a damaged piece of goods ever since I got sick'

- the *anger response*: it can be a great relief for patients to have anger acknowledged

- the *guilt response*: cancer may be seen as a punishment

- the *loss of gratification or pleasure*: for some, sexual gratification is lost as well

- the *response to the physician's attitude and behaviour*: patients' emotional responses to the disease and to the interventions of staff need to be treated as part of the problem.

Among the concerns of cancer patients are medical aspects, the accuracy of the diagnosis, the treatments and side-effects, and the prognosis; work and finances, occupation not only as a source of income but also of personal worth; family and significant relationships, a particular problem for those who are alone; sexual relationships and body image; and the effect of illness on the family. For some patients, existential concerns – thoughts about life and death – predominate (Weisman 1979a,b).

A number of first-person accounts of cancer patients have been published. They are an invaluable sourcebook for those who wish to understand the emotional side of the disease. One of the more memorable accounts is by Trillin (1981).

When I first realized that I might have cancer, I felt immediately that I had entered a special place, a place I came to call 'The Land of the Sick People' ... If I get sick, does that mean that my will to live isn't strong enough? Is being sick a moral and psychological failure? ... One of the ways that all of us avoid thinking about death is by concentrating on the details of our daily lives ... A year after I had my lung removed, my doctor asked me what I cared about most ... I told him that what was most important to me was garden peas ... What was extraordinary to me after that year was that I could again think that peas were important, that I could concentrate on the details of when to plant them and how much mulch they would need ... The strength of my love for my children, my husband, my life, even my garden peas has probably been more important than anything else in keeping me alive. The intensity of this love is also what makes me so terrified of dying ... We will never kill the dragon. But each morning we confront him. Then we give our children breakfast, perhaps put a bit more mulch on the peas, and hope that we can convince the dragon to stay away for a while longer.

Milton (1973) described 'thoughts in mind of a person with cancer'. In the early stage, fear dominated: fear of dying, of being dead and of leaving loved ones; fear of the effects of treatment and of loss of dignity; of mutilation; of revealing himself to be a coward (many attempts were made to conceal the terror); and suspicion of doctors and relatives, 'Are they telling me the truth?' Suspicion, he said, was based on fear. In the early stages the principal feelings were fear, doubt and suspicion, all of which fed one another. At a later stage, the 'Why me?' question arose, the natural response to which tends to be self-pity and resentment. In the final stages, when the cancer has recurred and the patient realises that attempts at cure have failed, a loneliness sets in:

Solzhenitzyn described the tumour as growing like a wall behind the patient; the patient's family and loved ones are on one side of the wall and the patient himself is alone on the other side ... The loneliness will also vary from time to time; during the day so long as the patient is in company and has something to occupy his mind he may well be able to suppress his loneliness, but at night, particularly if he has pain and the rest of the house is asleep, the feeling of isolation becomes almost overpowering.

One patient described the life issues that began to arise during the chronic phase of his disease: should he retire? sell his house? move into an apartment? leave the city to be nearer to family? During the terminal phase, he felt the need to have individual discussions with each of his children. Without using the word goodbye, it was basically to say a tentative goodbye (Papper 1985).

Some patients experience greater difficulty in coping with a cancer diagnosis than others. Weisman and Worden (1976–7) described what they termed the **existential plight** in cancer: the predictive significance for psychological adjustment of the first 100 days after diagnosis. The existential plight starts with diagnosis and continues for two to three months into the illness. Life/death concerns predominate at this time. Patients who had higher emotional distress during this period had many regrets about the past, were pessimistic, came from a multiproblem family or had marital problems. The widowed or divorced had higher vulnerability, as did patients who anticipated little or no support from significant others. These risk factors are an important guide to those patients who have the greatest need of counselling, as they are likely to be especially vulnerable not only in the 100 days following diagnosis, but as the disease progresses. Screening questions include:

Would you say that this illness has caused you to review and take stock of your life?

Would you say you have a lot of regrets about the past?

Do you think that, overall, you feel optimistic or pessimistic about the future?

Are there problems at home? In your relationship with your partner?

How many people are there who could look after you if you became seriously ill?

Patients who report mostly regrets about the past, who feel pessimistic about the future, who have problems at home and/ or in their most significant relationship and who have few if any friends or relations to look after them are vulnerable. Scarce counselling resources should be allocated to them, and more time will probably need to be given to them by medical and nursing staff in hospital. At each recurrence and relapse, and during palliative treatment and terminal care, some of the first reactions to illness may make a reappearance. It is as if fresh grief appears at every stage in some patients (Weisman 1979b).

The news of cancer triggers a **search for meaning** in the newly diagnosed patient (O'Connor *et al.*1990). Patients look for the personal significance of the diagnosis. Especially they have thoughts about what caused the cancer: 'Why has this happened to *me*?' They begin looking at the consequences of the cancer diagnosis on everyday activities, lifestyle and work, and to consider the possibility of death. There are the anticipated effects on those around them, including children who might inherit a predisposition to cancer. They review their lives, take stock, look back.

The patient may experience a change in outlook toward self, life and others. Some describe the diagnosis as a growing or learning experience. For others, there is a renewed appreciation of personal relationships or a strengthening of faith. As one patient put it, 'When something is taken away, you're given something back. And what was given back to me was family closeness. And if that's what it was, it was worth it'. Individuals may focus on the self, looking inward; or may look outward, in a renewed appreciation of nature: 'Taking more time to look at things, or listen, to watch the birds in the birdbath, just sit and listen to the wind chimes'. Many patients report a change in activities, doing things they have wanted to do for many years, such as creative work.

Cancer patients in the remission or recovery phase of cancer, when asked to describe its impact on their lives, focus on existential changes (Halldorsdottir and Hamrin 1996). Subthemes include uncertainty, vulnerability, isolation, discomfort and redefinition. Patients with different personality patterns are likely to find some of these more difficult than others. Those who need to be in control may find uncertainty and vulnerability most difficult. Others may feel intensely alone in their suffering, or cope poorly with pain. Still others may find their lives being redefined in ways they do not welcome. In particular, the state of suspended animation that follows the diagnosis has been described as 'living/dying' (Muzzin *et al.* 1994).

We can encourage cancer patients to describe their search for meaning as they come to terms with the disease. Useful interview questions include:

> In thinking about having cancer, what thoughts come into your mind?
>
> What has changed in your life since you discovered you have cancer?

Staff do not always have time to conduct an extended interview with the cancer patient at the time of diagnosis, but when there is time, some of the following questions may be useful. Not only do they allow the patient to tell the story of the illness, they also help the helper to anticipate future problems (Goldberg and Tull 1983).

How did you first become aware of your illness?

What made you finally decide to see a doctor?

What were your own ideas of what caused your symptoms?

How did you hear about your diagnosis?

What did the doctor tell you about the illness?

What did you feel when you heard the diagnosis?

When people receive upsetting news, they often find certain thoughts going through their minds over and over again. What recurring thoughts have you experienced?

How do you feel your partner has reacted to the diagnosis?

Who in your family has been hardest hit by this?

Is everyone in your family aware of the diagnosis?

How do you feel you will do with this illness? What do you see for yourself in the future?

Have you discussed your illness with your employer?

What has been the biggest problem since your diagnosis?

How much has your relationship with friends been affected?

Have any family or friends gone through a similar illness?

Have you ever been treated for a nervous condition? Has anyone in your family?

Do you see yourself as a religious person? Has there been a change since your diagnosis?

Have you spoken to clergy?

Prior to your present illness, what has been the biggest crisis you have had to face? What got you through that?

2
Cancer Treatments and Psychological Problems

Medical expertise is no guarantee of moral wisdom (Goldberg 1984).

Although people with cancer have in common the diagnosis of a life-threatening illness, many of the problems with which they struggle depend on the type and stage of their cancer and the treatment offered. Cancer follows a relatively predictable path – it has a natural history – and surgical or medical intervention is an attempt to stop progress along this path.

Disease Stage

The stage of a cancer is the extent to which it is restricted to the original tumour site: early stage (localized), limited spread to the original tumour area (loco-regional) or widely disseminated through the body (metastatic). Many cancers are diagnosed when the disease is a solid tumour confined to a single body site. An exception is a systemic disease such as leukaemia, which affects the blood. A small tumour confined to the breast may be more easily treated than a large tumour within the liver. Initial investigations attempt to ascertain the extent of spread from the tumour site to adjacent organs. As the disease becomes disseminated, major organs may fail. Some cancers are aggressive and carry a poorer prognosis because they are difficult to detect initially and are more often found only at a late stage. Factors influencing prognosis are complex and are influenced by the success of treatment. This is a large grey area, which makes it difficult for doctors to be specific about outcome. The wise doctor avoids putting a specific figure on a patient's life expectancy. Despite this, patients and their families sometimes grasp at these figures. It is quite common to hear a relative say, 'The doctor said he had six months'. Sometimes this happens because doctors feel they need to give a clear indication and will quote average figures for life expectancy at a given stage. However, these comments can be turned into a concrete figure by patients or relatives because inexactness is difficult to cope with and they may feel the need to deal with the situation in a concrete way. As the son of one patient put it:

> *I knew he was very ill. He was in the intensive care unit and his chances didn't seem good. I wanted the doctor to say whether he was going to pull through or die. I pursued this point every day with any doctor I could get hold of on the unit. None of them would say definitely. All they could say was that he was very ill, that his chances weren't good but that sometimes patients pulled through in this situation. This was no good for me. I needed to know ... the uncertainty was almost unbearable. Should I hope or should I grieve? Both seemed to be denied me in this situation.*

Cancer is a disease shot through with uncertainty, and it is this uncertainty that can make everything so stressful.

Cancer Treatments

Standard treatments for cancer fall into three main types: surgery, radiotherapy and chemotherapy. Surgery is usual where a solid tumour is confined to a single organ and where the aim is to remove this along with surrounding tissue before it has spread elsewhere. Radiotherapy is also used to destroy tumours before they have spread and to destroy any possibility of tumour cells arising around the site of the original tumour. It is also used when cancers have spread in order to relieve pain or discomfort. Chemotherapy is a systemic treatment, normally introduced into the blood in an attempt to destroy disseminated cancer cells.

Surgery is a brief intervention, radiotherapy is given over a period of a few weeks and chemotherapy over a few months. Chemotherapy is the most important development in cancer treatment and its role continues to change as new drugs are developed. For example, in breast cancer chemotherapy is increasingly used not only for disseminated disease but also to prevent disease spread. There are other treatments that are less commonly used and in some cases are experimental. The use of hormones in breast cancer has increased substantially since the mid-1980s. More recently, trials have begun using gene therapy, which manipulates the genetic structure of cells in such a way as to prevent further spread of malignancy. This area holds promise, but treatment trials are presently only at the threshold of progress in treating cancer.

This is a simplified description of a highly complex branch of medicine and is only intended to give a rough idea of the treatments used. Readers who are interested will find a substantial literature available to help them to gain a better understanding of the medical background to cancer treatment.

The Treatment Process

Treatment usually starts following the diagnosis, when people are first told they have a cancer. A description of the recommended treatments is often given at this point. The treatments themselves can be highly invasive, with toxic and unpleasant side effects such as nausea. Mutilating surgical procedures may be recommended, such as breast amputation. Treatments need to be implemented with the minimum of disruption to the patient's well-being and quality of life. For many patients whose disease is stable or in remission, the danger of relapse is always present and is an especially potent threat during the early months following diagnosis – the 'Damocles Syndrome' (Koocher and O'Malley 1981). The threat hangs like a sword over the patient's head; there is an unpredictability that will not go away. Should patients relapse, this can mean not only further treatment but also in many types of cancer it is often an indication that curative treatment is no longer possible. Therefore, relapse often signals to the patient that the sword has come down; it is the point of no return. It can confirm that the end of life is approaching. In some types of cancer, people go through this more than once. There is treatment, then remission, then relapse, and then it begins all over again: treatment, remission, relapse. This is especially demoralizing as patients slowly lose faith and suffer grave disappointment as they see their options disappearing.

For cancers that begin with solid tumours (as opposed to systemic diseases such as leukaemia) a relapse often indicates that the disease is spreading from the original tumour site to other parts of the body. This usually means further symptoms will arise. The type of symptom will depend on which parts of the body are affected. It is usually the process of metastasis that eventually kills people because vital organs begin to malfunction or shut down.

The dissemination of cancer to different parts of the body precedes the final and terminal stage where patients are dying. At this point, medical treatment is aimed solely at the palliation of symptoms. Prolongation of life is no longer a primary goal; the concern is to make the patient as comfortable as possible and to ease their dying. Patients and their families often find the process extremely confusing. They may not understand about their disease stage, why they are having a particular treatment and what to expect in the way of outcome or side effects. Medical terminology does not help; it mystifies the issues even more. Doctors and nurses need to be fully aware of the power of giving information. The impact of unclear information is illustrated by the following dialogue with a patient who had been treated for breast cancer:

> *Patient*: He (the doctor) told me in the hospital that he took my breast off because I didn't have cancer anywhere else in my body, I believed him ... but I'm on these tablets (tamoxifen) for two years, so that worries me. I think that I must be taking tablets because it's more likely that I'll get cancer again...
> *Interviewer*: Were you always worried about it coming back?
> *Patient*: No ... no ... no.... When he told me in the hospital that
>
> *continued*

continued

> he was going to take my breast off because I didn't have cancer in any other part of my body, and that I would have the medication for a while … Well, I understood that, but … he told me for two years I must have the tablets … I wonder why it's for two years that I have to take these tablets … That really worries me.

Psychological Aspects of Cancer Surgery

Many cancer patients undergo surgery. Staff who work daily on surgical wards can easily forget what a strange place it is, and it is a terrifying place to many patients. The intrusion of the scalpel into the body space violates a host of societal taboos, and the meaning of this intrusion to the individual patient may be important to uncover. In extreme cases, surgery may revive memories of trauma. For example, to a patient held in a prisoner of war camp, surgery may bring back unwanted memories or nightmares of torture. For survivors of sexual abuse, a hysterectomy may be the psychic equivalent of 'violence down below'. It is unfortunately not uncommon for women to remember childhood sexual abuse for the first time after pelvic surgery in their 40s, 50s or 60s.

To obsessional, tidy, or socially withdrawn people, the surgical ward can be a chamber of horrors that they find almost impossible to verbalize. People are losing limbs, drainage bottles hang from peoples' bodies discharging unpleasant fluids, patients are dying in the next bed and unwelcome operations are being performed on their own bodies about which they are often too frightened to ask even the most rudimentary questions. 'How do you feel about being in hospital for an operation?' is a useful way of asking about patients' fantasies about the surgical ward. Or, 'Some people find it difficult being on a surgical ward. How do you feel about being here for your operation?'

The patient must adjust to unfamiliar surroundings, hospital food and the sights, sounds and smells of the ward, operating theatre and recovery room. Some elderly people coming into hospital for cancer surgery may never have undergone an operation or been admitted to hospital before. The separation from home and from loved ones may be the most difficult feature for some of these patients. Occasionally, elderly patients will volunteer that this is the first time they have slept in a different bed from their partner. Such patients often need extra reassurance and support from staff during their hospital stay.

Fears of the anaesthetic are greater than fears of the operation for some patients. They may have many questions about the anaesthetic and may welcome being given an opportunity to voice their fears about general anaesthesia.

> Do you have any worries about being unconscious and not knowing what is going on?
>
> Any worries about waking up during the surgery, having any pain during the surgery, saying something embarrassing under the anaesthetic?
>
> Any worries about not waking up after the operation, about the masks or needles that the anaesthetist will use?
>
> Would you say that you are more afraid of the anaesthetic than you are of the operation?

For needle phobics, starting an intravenous drip and undergoing anaesthesia may be the most difficult features of their hospitalization. Claustrophobic patients, especially among the elderly, may believe that they will be given 'gas' to breathe and they may find the idea of a mask over their face frightening. The prospect of being trapped on an operating table unable to control what is going on may be especially difficult for these patients. People who are frightened before surgery almost always welcome an opportunity to verbalize their fears and receive information and appropriate reassurance from hospital staff.

Some patients are most frightened of postoperative pain. Others are more worried about the outcome of the operation. They may be asking, 'Will surgery help? Will more be needed later on?'. This is especially the case when the surgery is exploratory or palliative. For some, fears of dying are paramount, especially if a relative died of the same disease or following the same operation. There is an important difference between the patient who fears death and the patient who calmly predicts death as a result of the operation. Those who announce that they will die during the operation have, as one surgeon put it, 'a very nasty tendency to do just that'. They are high risk and surgery may need to be postponed in order to work through the underlying psychological issues (Boehnert 1986).

Surgery carries with it the risk of postoperative depression or (much more rarely) postoperative psychosis. Many patients find that as long as they are supported in hospital and later in the radiotherapy or chemotherapy department they make good progress, but many report severe depression setting in after the surgery and adjuvant treatments have finished. A number of patients feel suddenly abandoned by the health care team, and the general practitioner has a vital role to play at this time. Support groups for patients with certain kinds of cancer may also help to protect against postoperative depression (Chapter 11). In some patients, antidepressant medication is indicated, especially when there has been a preoperative history of psychiatric illness.

To many, surgery for cancer can be expected to bring death. To some, having cancer surgery is evidence of punishment. To a few, cancer is something that should be allowed to take its course, and these patients welcome news of a sooner-than-expected end to a miserable life. To others, it is something to fight, a challenge, something to overcome. Cancer may be seen as the alien eating away at the self from within, 'cells out of control', or something dirty and shameful. 'When you think about the word cancer, what comes to mind?' is a good first question to find out how the patient feels about the disease.

The *meaning* of the organ or organ system to the patient is important, especially when organ loss is a factor. One of the psychological tasks during a stay on a surgical ward may be grieving for the loss of an important body part. Here, past experiences of grieving may predict the patient's response to the present loss. 'What has been the biggest loss you had to face prior to this operation?' is a helpful question, with the follow-up, 'And what got you through that?' Those patients who responded to earlier losses with helplessness, hopelessness and suicidal ideas may find the present loss even more difficult to negotiate and may need to be referred for psychotherapy. Some patients have experienced a combination of stressful life events of which the diagnosis of cancer is only the most recent (Chapters 7 and 8).

The loss of a limb, part of the face, larynx, a breast, the rectum or any of the reproductive organs (uterus, ovaries, vagina, vulva, testicles, penis) is particularly traumatic, and these patients have special needs. Two of the commonest but most mutilating cancer operations are mastectomy (removal of the breast) and colostomy (excision of the rectum and the creation of an artificial opening on the abdomen that discharges faeces into a bag). Because these operations cause so many psychological and psychosexual complications, they are discussed separately in Chapter 5. Surgery for cancer of the genitalia carries similar high risks for complications.

The loss of facial features in head and neck cancers, even when prostheses are available, is deeply traumatic to virtually every patient because the face presents the self to the world more than any other body part. Laryngectomy, even when appliances make it possible for some sound to be made, is similarly traumatic because of the damage to the ability to communicate. But the *meaning* of the organ that is lost must be discovered anew with each individual patient. Loss of the breast to a young, sexually active, attractive divorced woman may be experienced as a major catastrophe while the same operation in an elderly widow is accepted philosophically. Similarly, a colostomy may be accepted by an elderly patient in a way that it is not by a younger person. Loss of a limb in a young runner, laryngectomy in a lecturer, mastectomy in a gymnast or ballet dancer – these will obviously be traumatic; yet the meaning of the loss of the body part may be quite unexpected and specific to a given patient. It is important that helpers do not jump to conclusions until they have spoken in depth with the patient about it. An open-ended question may help: 'When you think about losing your [breast], what thoughts and feelings come to mind about it?'

There are a number of mediating factors that affect patients' responses to cancer surgery. **Coping style** will be discussed in the next chapter, where we examine the special problems posed by denial. The patient's **social support network** has been shown to predict adjustment to surgery. Similarly, **stressful life events** may have a predictive impact on adjustment, especially when the patient has undergone a number of previous stressors in the preceding months or years. **Personality type** (Chapter 1) may have an important impact on adjustment to cancer surgery. Psychologists often speak of a patient's **ego strength**, by which they mean inner resources in the face of external stress. **Past response to loss or stress** is another good predictor of outcome. High-risk surgical patients are those with

- poor social support, few or no relatives and no one to look after them at home

- many recent stressful life events prior to the diagnosis

- poor ego strength

- a history of psychological collapse in the face of previous loss or stress

- personality styles that involve an unstable or brittle set of defences (dependent, compulsive, hysterical, masochistic, narcissistic, schizoid and paranoid, see Chapter 1).

In the initial interview with the surgeon, patients have many concerns about surgery, but some of these are rarely addressed by the consultant. Sometimes the assumption is made that junior doctors or nursing staff will attend to these issues later on in hospital. Often enough, however, questions continue to go unanswered and preoperative worries mount. Questions that often go unanswered in the initial consultation include the cause of the disease, the effects of the surgery on sexual functioning, the psychological side effects of the surgery, the anaesthetic and postoperative pain, the impact of the operation on the family, practical support at home, where the patient will be when coming round from the anaesthetic, how soon the patient will be able to get out of bed or eat a meal, who will actually do the surgery and the operative risk (Burton and Parker 1997).

Effects of Radiotherapy and Chemotherapy

For many cancer patients, the trauma does not end with surgery. Indeed for many it is just beginning because the emotional impact of radiotherapy and chemotherapy can be considerable, and these may come at a time when the patient feels unready for any new stress. Eardley (1985) has described patients' reactions to radiotherapy:

> *They put the lights out and out they went – they ran for the door. You didn't know what the hell was going to happen.*
> *It's like going into a strange land – that machine looks like something from outer space.*
> *They just said I'd get a sore mouth - I didn't know how sore.*
> *They tell you what to expect but they don't tell you about this weakness.*
> *The staff say you'll be over the worst in a month, so it comes as a bit of a shock when at two months you're still feeling pretty low.*

The provision of information can make a positive impact in the case of both chemotherapy and radiotherapy (Ream and Richardson 1996). BACUP has produced excellent booklets on these treatments, as well as one on coping with hair loss, a common side effect (BACUP 1994a,b,c). They have also published a very useful set of booklets explaining a wide range of cancers to the general public. Many patients report that reading a booklet about radiotherapy makes the treatment seem less frightening and helps them feel more confident. The booklet informs patients that marks will probably be made on their skin to pinpoint where the radiation will be directed. A see-through mould for their head and neck may be made if irradiation must be given to that area. Internal radiotherapy (radioactive implants) is explained along with the need for an inpatient stay, visitor restrictions and lead shields. Side effects of radiotherapy are described, including blood changes necessitating regular tests, painful mouth, loss of appetite and weight loss, voice changes, hair loss, difficulty in swallowing, nausea and vomiting, shortness of breath, diarrhoea, pain while passing urine, tiredness and skin reactions. Radiotherapy to the ovaries will cause the menopause. The vagina may be narrowed when it is irradiated. Men undergoing radiotherapy may have loss of libido or become temporarily impotent through anxiety. Radiotherapy to the ovaries or testes can lead to temporary or permanent sterility.

Abnormal psychological reactions to radiotherapy may occur when special meaning is attached to the treatment. For example, some patients believe that radiotherapy is offered only when nothing else can be done. When life events compound the situation, for example a recent bereavement, a patient may have no wish to live and show little interest in treatment for his/her own carcinoma. Fear of being trapped under the machine may be a problem, for example in a man who had narrowly escaped death pinned under a car. In cases of prior history of severe agoraphobia, panic attacks, paranoid personality disorder or schizophrenia, liaison with a psychiatrist or clinical psychologist may be very important (Holland 1989).

Similarly, chemotherapy may cause a host of side effects, principally nausea and vomiting. Patients can begin to be nauseous or vomit when thinking about the hospital, when approaching the building or when walking onto the ward. This **anticipatory nausea and vomiting** can be treated behaviourally by a clinical psychologist. Regular blood tests will usually be made to assess damage to the bone marrow. Resistance to infection often decreases and antibiotics may be prescribed. Hair loss is one of the most distressing side effects of chemotherapy, and fatigue will have generally debilitating effects not only during the treatment but, in some patients, for many months after (Cull 1990). Patients undergoing radiotherapy or chemotherapy need an opportunity to discuss the side effects of the treatment, their experiences in the oncology unit and their feelings about the procedure. Counselling at these stages of treatment needs to give patients space to describe their feelings and work them through.

Bone Marrow Transplant and Hormonal Therapies

Bone marrow transplantation is now an important treatment for haematological malignancies, but the procedure places patients under severe psychological stress (Lesko 1993a,b). Patients are in isolation to avoid infection and it is a stressful time for the family. Children may find the isolation ward and the appearance of a loved parent frightening. Pretransplant conditioning may include high-dose immunosuppressive drugs and total body irradiation. A Hickman catheter is inserted under local anaesthesia in order that blood samples may be easily drawn and medications given. High-dose chemotherapy is then administered to destroy the existing bone marrow.

The early days of the procedure are marked by anxiety alternating with hope, and episodes of nausea, vomiting and fatigue occur secondary to the irradiation and chemotherapy. The transplant is administered rapidly in an infusion. The possibilities of infection and/or graft-versus-host disease raise anxieties at the post-transplant stage. Discharge may not occur for one or two months. Many patients become regressed, suffer depression and anxiety, or reject treatment when the stress of the procedure becomes too great. Convalescence can last up to six months. Bone marrow transplant is a high-risk procedure, and survival is not guaranteed. Some patients undertake it with only a 50–50 chance of survival. The procedure tends to be used in patients with severe or life-threatening disease.

Hormonal treatments, for example tamoxifen for breast cancer, tend to cause less psychological morbidity than radiotherapy, chemotherapy or bone marrow transplant, but the side effects in individual patients can be considerable. Hot flushes, irregular vaginal bleeding and nausea are common side effects of tamoxifen, and some patients become depressed. Some hormonal treatments for cancer cause menstrual periods to cease, the growth of body hair and a masculinized voice in women, and impotence and breast enlargement in men. Hormonal therapy for metastatic prostate cancer, with the goal of reducing testosterone levels to zero, impairs sexual desire. Men on hormonal therapy also often have difficulty achieving erection or reaching orgasm. Steroids can cause pronounced mood changes (especially elation) and bodily changes such as a moon-shaped face and weight gain. All of these changes affect feelings of well-being and may markedly affect sexual function.

Psychological Problems

Problems of adjustment are common in people undergoing cancer treatment. Cancer patients are essentially normal people going through abnormal stress and are, by and large, not suffering from psychiatric disorders. The major problems are usually an adjustment disorder with anxiety and/or depression. Research suggests that anxiety is the most common form of distress (Watson *et al.* 1991; Greer *et al.* 1992) and this is especially so during the few weeks following diagnosis, recurrence or spread. Other psychological effects include sexual and marital dysfunction (Reiker *et al.* 1985; Moynihan 1987; Wellisch *et al.* 1992), treatment-related problems such as nausea and vomiting occurring as a conditioned side-effect of chemotherapy (Andrykowski *et al.* 1988; Watson *et al* 1992), steroid-induced psychiatric disorders (Lewis and Smith 1983; Mitchell and Collins 1984) and problems in social and occupational functioning. The pattern of 'abnormal illness behaviour' (high levels of hypochondriasis, a conviction that the cancer has spread when it has not, low mood and irritability) has been linked to a lifetime history of psychiatric disorder or a present psychiatric disorder. Poor social support also contributes to this picture (Grassi and Rosti 1996).

Coping with cancer pain can be exacerbated by mental state, with depressed and anxious patients being more likely to report pain or pain-related problems. Turk and Fernandez (1991) have argued eloquently that although cancer pain usually has a clear physical basis there are psychological elements to pain perception, suggesting that helping patients to cope with pain may involve the use of psychological methods. Above all, this should include more effective communication to dispel some of the myths and fears surrounding cancer pain and the methods available to control it.

The impact of cancer diagnosis and treatment on daily life and the patient's ability to carry on working can be far-reaching and may cause significant problems. Moynihan (1987) discussed the impact of cancer treatment on employment for men with testicular cancer. She found that 46% of men who were treated for this cancer and were unemployed at any time over the period after their treatment had psychological problems, compared with 14% of those who had been continuously in work. Financial strain was found to be significantly associated with psychological stress and unemployment in these patients.

The most common feeling experienced by people with cancer is anxiety. People also report a range of other problems including irritability, sleep disturbance, inability to concentrate, loss of appetite, loss of sexual interest, and tiredness and lethargy, which are not necessarily treatment or disease related but are symptoms of stress. Depression and feelings of helplessness and hopelessness are also common. These can arise directly as a result of dealing with the disease and also from the disruption to normal activities that can occur while people are on treatment.

Mrs. A was receiving treatment for breast cancer that involved regular infusions of chemotherapy drugs. The chemotherapy made her feel tired and sick. She worried that it might not be helping or even that it might be harming her (*anxiety*). Because she felt so unwell after her chemotherapy she could not see how it would be doing her any good. She began to think that it was inevitable the cancer would come back and that it was only a matter of time before this happened (*hopelessness*). When she was at home she often felt overwhelmed by worries that the cancer would come back (*anxious preoccupation*) or even that it already had, but the doctors had missed it on the tests. She stopped going out to meet her girlfriends for coffee as she used to and no longer felt like doing things around the house. Some mornings she did not feel like getting up and seemed to drift through the day (*depression*). Then she would feel terrible because so much time had been wasted with nothing having been done (*guilt*).

As the time for the next hospital visit drew nearer she became more and more tense and worried. Her husband found her irritable and difficult. She was aware of this but did not seem able to do anything about it (*helplessness*). This made her feel worse, and to add to her other worries she began to feel that she might drive him away (*guilt*). When she was due to go for her next chemotherapy she got extremely wound up. She arrived at the hospital, but because she began to feel sick, she went home without having her next cycle of chemotherapy. This exacerbated her worry because if she missed or delayed the chemotherapy she thought the cancer would

continued

continued

definitely not be cured. During the following two or three nights she could not sleep because of the intolerable level of anxiety.

What could she do? (*helplessness*) She did not want to go to hospital, but she did not want to die. She bottled all of this up because she had not been getting along well with her husband and felt unable to talk to him about it. She now neglected her appearance and her housework. There was increasing tension between her and her husband.

Suicide Risk

Occasionally cancer patients become so severely depressed that they are suicidal. *When this occurs, it is advisable to request a psychiatric assessment as a matter of urgency.* On the one hand, the patient who becomes deeply withdrawn may be contemplating suicide. On the other hand some patients known to be depressed become unaccountably cheerful after having taken the decision to end their life, with a lethal plan in mind. Staff need to be alert for hints that suicide is being considered:

If only I could fall asleep and it would all be over
I don't think I can bear this much longer
There's no point in going on.

Such hints should be followed up with a risk assessment: does the patient have a plan, how lethal is that plan, under what circumstances might they carry it out and how likely does the patient think it is that they will act on the plan? Patients at greater risk of suicide have a previous history of suicide attempts, have suffered a recent loss (such as bereavement or redundancy), are socially isolated and experience chronic problems such as housing or financial difficulties (Faulkner and Maguire 1996).

Patients At Risk of Psychological Problems

Factors associated with increased distress are:

- a previous psychiatric history

- lack of support from family and friends

- inability to accept the physical changes associated with the disease or its treatment

- lack of involvement in satisfying activities

- a prior adverse experience of cancer in the family

- low expectations regarding the effectiveness of treatment

- pre-existing marital problems

- younger age at diagnosis.

Social support is an important predictor of health in its own right. Separated and divorced people are at higher risk than those who are happily married, or those who are well adjusted to single life or widow(er)hood with good extended support networks. Social support can be a stress as well as a buffer: when marital quality is poor, for example, it is a source of added stress. When the support network provides emotional sustenance, helps with problem solving and provides the commitment of a continuing alliance, it can have a powerful buffering effect against psychological problems associated with cancer. Effective social support systems may improve length of survival (Creagan 1997).

Age, support systems and level of prediagnostic functioning appear to have an important impact on coping ability and level of adjustment (Weisman 1979a; Bloom 1982; Hughes 1982; Dean 1987). For a more comprehensive review of psychosocial problems, the reader is directed to Holland and Rowland's (1989) excellent book, which provides a wide-ranging review of the problems commonly encountered.

Common Themes to Patients' Problems

There are a number of themes to patients' problems and these underlie some of the observed difficulties. Often the initial diagnosis is accompanied by a feeling of shock. Feelings of anger may quickly follow and frequently people will ask, 'Why me, what did I do to deserve this?' Some people blame themselves not only for getting the disease but also for the suffering it causes their families. Some feel a deep sense of shame at having cancer, which can lead to social isolation and an inability to communicate their feelings.

Some patients are totally unprepared for the diagnosis because they were unaware of any symptoms suggesting they were ill. In breast cancer, for example, the woman often has no prior symptoms and indeed may feel quite well. With the discovery of a malignant tumour, in an instant she becomes a patient with a life-threatening disease. This can cause feelings of confusion and loss of control. For many people the diagnosis means uncertainty about the future.

Will I see my children grow up?
Will I be able to enjoy the retirement I planned?
Will I be able to carry on with my job?

Uncertainty can bring feelings of helplessness, often expressed as not being able to do anything to change the course of the disease. This feeling of futility and of not knowing where to turn or what to do to try to change events was expressed by the wife of one patient: 'We are like goldfish going round and round in a bowl with no way out'. Those who were previously in control of their lives now find it to be out of control.

There may be a fear of dying, 'Will it be painful?', 'What will it be like?', 'What will happen?', 'How will I die?'; and resistance, 'I am not ready to die', 'I don't deserve to die', I am too young, I haven't done all the things I want to do yet'. These feelings can be closely linked to existential issues around whether life has been fulfilling. Sometimes people are able to come to terms with the threat of death by saying, 'I've had a good life, what's left is a bonus', whereas others question whether they have been conducting their lives as they should. Regrets may surface and cloud their ability to gain pleasure from the remaining months of their life. As one patient put it, 'I've done a lot of things I regret, and it hasn't always been easy for my family. I wish I could change things. I feel that

I've wasted my life'. These existential issues are illustrated by the character Ursula in David Lodge's book *Paradise News* (1991). She has been told that she has disseminated malignant melanoma and therefore a very limited life expectancy. She quips to her nephew who is visiting her:

> *I've done nothing with my life. What could they put on my tombstone? 'She played a mean game of bridge'. 'At 69 she could still swim a half a mile'. 'Her chocolate fudge was very popular'. That's about it.*

Some people may be filled with regrets and can feel very depressed that the things they want for themselves still lie in the future unfulfilled, and that cancer is denying or cheating them of opportunities. For younger patients there is a special poignancy to the often expressed regret that they will not see their children grow up to adulthood. When a loss is sustained without resolution in a chronic and life-threatening situation, a state of 'chronic sorrow' may result (Hainsworth *et al.* 1994).

Cancer often brings a loss of dignity because of physical changes brought about by the disease or its treatment. These may result, for example, from the need to have a colostomy to allow the removal of faeces from the body, from the hair loss that accompanies chemotherapy, or the vomiting that occurs as a side effect of cytotoxic drugs. Affected parts of the body may need to be surgically removed, and this mutilation may be visible to others. A leg may be removed because of a sarcoma (a cancer that affects the muscle or bone). Other tumours may necessitate the removal of a breast or part of the face. These have an impact on body image and repercussions for a person's self-esteem. As one woman put it:

> *I wish it (the operation scar) wasn't there, that's all ... I wouldn't let anybody see me without my clothes on. I just look at myself in the mirror and I think ... Oh God! Men wouldn't find me attractive ... not with this scar ... I don't think so anyway.*

Cancer may cause weight loss and a gradual wasting of muscles. These can all contribute to loss of dignity and in some instances to a profound loss of self-esteem or self-confidence. People who previously thought they were in control of their lives can find the situation drastically changed, and it can be hard to maintain self-esteem and self-confidence in such circumstances.

Another common theme involves the inability to tolerate treatment. Noncompliance with treatment is common among patients who could benefit substantially, and this can sometimes be prevented by sensitive counselling. Given the number of distressing side effects of cancer treatments and the risk that a remission or cure will not be forthcoming (especially in the case of experimental treatments), it is not surprising that some patients decide they do not wish to proceed with treatment. It is important to avoid undue pressure on the patient who has come to a decision after being fully informed of the consequences, and to respect such decisions once they have been made. In some American centres, an ethics consultant may be available or a hospital chaplain may help to mediate between patient and medical staff. Psychology staff may be called in to consult, particularly outside the USA.

Cancers are essentially chronic diseases, and treatment can continue over long periods with side effects ranging from the irritating to the debilitating. Where patients hope for cure they are often prepared to endure the treatments, although even then lengthy periods of treatment can become difficult to tolerate. Where treatment is not curative but is aimed at buying time, they can become demoralized by toxic side effects. They may not know whether the treatment will give them more time, because it is difficult for clinicians to say what can be expected. They may become depressed when they cannot enjoy the time they have left. In such circumstances the treatment is often perceived as worse than the disease. If the patient is depressed, such thoughts may be part of their depression. However, it should not be assumed that patients expressing this view are always clinically depressed. When quality of life is poor, it may not be an unrealistic view. This problem is perhaps more common than is widely acknowledged. Fortunately, in a substantial number of cases it is possible to review treatment, look at other options and obtain better control over side effects, as in the case of Mrs W.

Mrs W was being treated for cancer of the bowel and she had been receiving chemotherapy, not to cure the disease but to prolong her life. This involved regular injections of cytotoxic drugs over a period of months. One particular drug caused her to experience extreme lethargy. As a consequence, she was unable to carry on her normal domestic activities. She had a history of depressive illness that may have increased her vulnerabilty. Losing her ability to maintain usual daily patterns caused her to feel depressed and she lost confidence in her ability to look after her husband and carry on as normal. The depression contributed further by reducing her motivation ('It's not worth trying') and locked her into a cycle she felt unable to break. The depression worsened and she began to express suicidal ideas.

Some patients are able to balance the costs and benefits of a noncurative treatment and decide it has been worthwhile. If they feel it has not produced the benefits they anticipated, they may become frustrated or depressed. They may get angry about the time wasted on trying to cope with the side effects of invasive medical and surgical treatments that in the end have brought only a few extra months of life. When patients decide that their quality of life is unacceptably poor with treatment and they prefer to spend the short time left to them at home with their families, this decision may be in conflict with the health care team's treatment plan. A few doctors are over-zealous in promoting treatment at the expense of quality of life. At other times, the patient has unrealistic expectations of what will happen if they discontinue treatment. If patients say they wish to opt out of or stop treatment, it becomes important to determine whether this is a fully informed decision or whether it is based on purely emotional concerns (Faulkner and Maguire 1996).

3
Coping with Cancer

Coping is an attempt to ward off, reduce or assimilate a stressor, either through ways of thinking and feeling or by taking action (Heim 1991). Therefore, adjustment to cancer is defined by the cognitive, emotional and behavioural responses people make to the diagnosis. Considerable distress is associated with cancer and there is evidence that the type of coping response invoked is an important contributor to these difficulties (Altmaier *et al.* 1982; Nerenz *et al.* 1982; Parle *et al.* 1994).

Psychological problems may be greater where the patient's coping response involves fatalism, displacement or projection. Everson *et al.* (1996) found hopelessness to be associated with significantly increased risk. Watson *et al.* (1984) found denial to be associated with less distress, while, in another study, fighting spirit and emotional expressiveness were associated with better adjustment (Classen *et al.* 1996). It is important to understand the ways in which people cope with cancer. A prerequisite of good communication is to know how patients are thinking and feeling. Lack of insight into how patients or relatives are coping with the disease can be a recipe for disaster when it comes to communicating effectively.

Styles of Coping

Greer *et al.* (1979) described a number of coping styles among women with breast cancer.

- Fighting spirit. The tendency to see the illness as a challenge and to strive to prevent it from overwhelming them: 'I believe that my positive attitude will benefit my health'.

- Helplessness. The tendency to feel utterly at a loss and unable to do anything about the impact that cancer has upon their lives: 'I feel the situation is hopeless'.

- Stoic acceptance. The tendency to view things in a passive way and accept things for what they are: 'There's nothing you can do about it'.

- Denial. The tendency to block from conscious awareness anything associated with the threat: 'I don't really believe I had a cancer'.

These categories have been subsequently modified in the light of more recent research (Watson *et al.* 1994) and additional coping styles have been identified.

- Anxious preoccupation. The tendency to focus on having cancer, allowing the disease to dominate life, thereby increasing anxiety; searching daily for new lumps.

- Fatalism. The tendency to accept things for what they are and make no attempt to take control; passivity in the face of disease and the treatments offered: 'It's in others' hands'.

- Cognitive avoidance. The tendency to find ways of avoiding thoughts or blocking off worrying feelings. This differs from denial in that patients may be conscious of the fact that they are avoiding thinking about cancer.

These categories do not represent every coping response but provide a basis for understanding how patients set about coping with cancer. Some simple questions asked within the context of history-taking may help to clarify the person's usual coping strategy.

Fighting spirit: 'Is taking a positive attitude something that is difficult or easy for you?'

Helplessness: 'It's not unusual to feel overwhelmed and helpless. How do you feel about what has happened?'

Stoic acceptance: 'Some people feel they want to leave everything to the doctor. Is that how you feel?'

Denial: see below

Anxious preoccupation: 'It sounds like you've been seeking a lot of information about your illness. Has this helped or do you think it makes you worry more?'

Fatalism: 'Are you the sort of person who tends to accept things as they are or do you question what goes on?'

Cognitive avoidance: 'Some people find it helps to avoid thinking about things to do with their illness. Are you that sort of person?'

Denial as a Response to Cancer

Some coping responses that may be encountered when dealing with cancer patients pose specific problems. The use of denial or avoidance is a commonly encountered reaction that causes some disagreement among professionals. The main issue arises from whether or not it is adaptive and, if not, how it should be challenged.

It is easy to fall into the trap of believing that all patients at some point need to talk about what has happened to them or how they are feeling. **Ventilation of emotions** is a focal element in counselling but caution is needed here. People who are very uncomfortable talking about deep emotions and fears may never broach the issues; indeed, they often refuse to do so. The simplest way to deal with this is to ask if they want to talk about what is on their mind and not to press ahead and assume that they must want to talk about any worries. The communication process should always allow the patient the option to avoid discussion of challenging topics. However, there is sometimes pressure from either family or staff for the patient to acknowledge their plight. It is possible as a helper to find oneself in the situation where doctors, nurses or a spouse have asked that the patient be counselled only to find that the patient becomes extremely uncomfortable because they cannot bear to talk about their fears.

What is Denial?

True denial, in the psychoanalytic sense, is rare among people with cancer. It involves a total blocking out of what is happening. Patients who show this response may go so far as to deny that surgical scars exist, or may insist that they are being treated for a minor ailment; a patient with an enormous fungating breast tumour applies creams and dressings and does not present for help until it is bleeding and oozing through the skin. Another patient explains bone metastases as the result of a fall from a ladder. More frequently it is not the denial of the symptoms or diagnosis that occurs, but a denial of the emotional impact of the illness (Wool and Goldberg 1986).

Patients who use denial show a benign reaction to all that is going on around them and may produce complex explanations for what is happening to them. For example, a patient who has been told he has cancer, when asked for his own understanding of what is wrong, says, 'I don't know, I just have this pain in my chest'. In psychoanalytic terms this represents an unconscious disavowal of any threat. It is this unconscious element that distinguishes denial from the far more common response among cancer patients of avoidance. The primary element that distinguishes denial from avoidance is the absence, in the denying patient, of overt symptoms of anxiety or depression. The denying patient frequently presents a bland countenance and holds a completely unrealistic view of events, for example, 'I'm going to be fine', despite declining strength and widely disseminated disease. Patients who respond with avoidance may indeed suffer some distress but are struggling to exclude the stressful issues from conscious awareness. They often have a realistic view of their disease and are frightened by it.

Avoidance and denial may operate at a number of levels (Watson 1984). There may be avoidance of the physical symptoms, with an attempt to hide the fact that a lump exists. Often this response can be related to delay in seeking treatment for advanced disease. This is quite rare now, as people have become more aware that early diagnosis is essential to successful treatment. Denial of the diagnosis of cancer is somewhat more common, for example, 'The doctor just took my breast off as a precaution'. More frequent, however, is avoidance of the implications of cancer, for example, 'It's only a few bad cells, it isn't really serious'. Finally there is avoidance of feelings, with the patient admitting the diagnosis but denying that they are distressed by it, although careful probing may reveal they are actually deeply distressed (Greer 1992).

It is important when attempting to establish if patients are using denial or avoidance to check the following:

- exclude organic brain syndrome and psychotic illness
- establish what the patient has actually been told, as patients cannot avoid or deny things for which they have no knowledge in the first place
- establish how long it is since they were told the diagnosis.

Avoidance can be very common as an initial response to the diagnosis, but this often changes rapidly and is replaced by other emotional reactions such as anger, guilt and anxiety. Persistent avoidance is quite rare; more often it fluctuates, with distress breaking through from time to time.

Dealing with Denial and Avoidance

Denial has often been considered a poor coping response and one that predisposes the patient to delay in mentioning further symptoms. This is possible, but more usually it is a strategy that people adopt when they feel overwhelmed by events and emotions; it can be a very effective way of helping them to gain some relief from their anxiety or depression.

When deciding how to deal with avoidance, there is a good argument for leaving well alone unless patients give some indication that they are not sustaining the positive effects of that coping strategy, or that they do indeed want to think about the issues at another point in time, if the situation changes. It is such a powerful psychological response that it can be quite difficult to challenge. If there is a request to counsel patients who are avoiding the issues of their cancer, the most telling indication of whether to respond lies quite simply in who asks for this help. It is hardly ever the patient and is more likely to be a familiy member or a member of the nursing or medical team. It is they who are uncomfortable with the idea that the implications of the cancer diagnosis are being avoided.

Minimizing the threat of cancer is a way of coping with something that otherwise would be emotionally over-whelming. Patients have been known to maintain this avoidance reaction up to the point of their death. Avoidance can be an effective method of keeping powerful unpleasant emotions at bay. It can also be a strategy for maintaining a positive attitude toward the disease. It is difficult to maintain hope for the future if evidence shows that you will soon die. For some people, it is the only way to get through on a day-to-day basis, and so there can be a time when avoidance is appropriate. The problem for staff working with people with cancer is to know how to test subtly whether there is evidence of positive avoidance and if this is beneficial to the patient.

Some people will indicate that they realise the situation is serious but will then quickly give the message that they have filed this knowledge away and no further discussion is necessary. Any attempt to break this down could result in the disintegration of the relationship that has been formed with the patient. It is important to make a person aware that the door is always open should they feel the need to talk. Successful denial or avoidance reduces distress. Where distress is evident, then it may be more helpful gently to encourage the person to talk about their concerns.

For many of the nursing and medical staff the issue is clouded by the need to push forward treatments for the disease in those patients who may be denying its threat. Frequently the worry revolves around the patient's possible noncompliance with recommended treatments. It is possible, however, to explain the need for treatment in a way that allows patients to maintain their defence. The ultimate threat, 'If you don't have this treatment you're going to die', is likely to be perceived exactly as a threat, and the recommended treatment plan may be resisted. An alternative is to ask:

Would you like to know more about the treatment options?

To what extent would you like to be involved in the decisions about your medical treatment?

Do you need more time to think about the treatment options before the decision is made?

Do you have any particular worries about the treatment we've been discussing?

Do you want to know any more about why this particular treatment has been recommended?

Denial or avoidance may have an adaptive function, but in some circumstances it can be maladaptive. The task for the doctor or others working with patients is to determine which it might be in current circumstances before deciding how to proceed.

Dealing with Anger

Some people cope with cancer by ventilating their anger. Being the target of patients' anger is one of the most difficult situations in cancer care. It is often unexpected. More often than not patients behave towards those caring for their health in a socially acceptable way, indeed often with a feeling of gratitude, so it can come as something of a shock to have to cope with hostile or aggressive emotions. Despite this, it is probably true to say that all professions working with cancer patients will at some time find themselves on the receiving end of someone's anger. It is important to accept that this will happen from time to time, to understand why it can happen and to know how to deal with it.

Not surprisingly, the first reaction to being at the sharp end of an angry reaction is to defend ourselves and explain our actions if it seems we have done something to cause this anger. Anger is not an uncommon emotional reaction but because of social pressures people usually keep such feelings to themselves. Patients may be frustrated and angry about getting cancer; the feeling of 'Why me?' They may be angry because where once they were in control of their lives, now they have to face something that is out of their control. They also become part of the health care system and may feel in a position of weakness. They may have to put up with long periods of waiting for results, waiting to see doctors and a host of other seemingly unnecessary delays. They may be afraid and insecure.

When a patient or relative becomes angry, it is important to find out why this is happening. A good first principle in facing anger from patients is not to try to defend one's actions, because to do so has the effect of sucking you into the conflict by becoming part of it and creating an escalating situation. Instead it helps to acknowledge the anger, to give the person an opportunity to make their point and then to say 'Okay, what can we do about this?' Allow them to express the angry feelings first, and then the person will be better able to be more rational. Always the aim is to see beyond the personal attack in order to discern if a solution is possible. Done the right way you move from being the person's adversary to being their ally, as demonstrated in the case of Mrs A.

Mrs A was admitted in order to have a bone marrow transplant. This is a risky procedure made more difficult by the fact that the patient commonly spends a few weeks in isolation being barrier nursed in order to reduce the risk of infection. Before admission, she was given a locker in which she could keep her personal belongings. The whole admission procedure was anxiety-provoking for her. Upon opening the locker she found some mouldy items of food left by a previous patient. She complained to the nurse about the dirty state of the locker. The nurse explained that the locker had become free only that morning. It was normally the responsibility of patients or their families to clear the lockers, but the previous patient's family had failed to do this because they were upset at her death the night before. Mrs A then rounded on the nurse angrily, saying she had behaved in a totally unprofessional way by mentioning that the person had died.

She then complained about a host of other irritating events: the length of time they had kept her waiting to be admitted, the lack of information about what she was supposed to do. In this instance, the nurse could have leapt to her own defence. However, she recognized that it was mentioning the death of the previous patient that was the key to the patient's anger, and she asked Mrs A to accompany her to a side room. The patient continued her angry outburst and threatened to report the nurse to her superiors. In response the nurse accepted that Mrs A was feeling very angry; she apologized for mentioning the death of the previous patient and suggested that it may have frightened Mrs A to hear it put so

continued

continued

bluntly. She went on to ask the patient about how she felt about coming into hospital and then gently encouraged her to express her own fears.

In this way the patient was able to say, privately and in her own time, that she was extremely frightened about the bone marrow transplant and had found it hard to face the idea that she might die. She had felt unable to confide this to her family for fear of upsetting them. They were then able to talk about what it was that she feared and went on to explore how she might develop ways of coping with the impending procedure. Had the nurse reacted defensively in this instance, the eventual outcome would have been of little help to all concerned.

The urge to defend one's position is strong but needs to be resisted if anger is to be dealt with and the patient is to be allowed to express this strong emotion.

Anger may be perceived as an unacceptable emotion in some patients and is then expressed in other forms, for example as symptom distress or depression (Taylor *et al.* 1993). It is well known clinically that anger can be the principal underlying dynamic in severe depression.

4
Family Issues

Cancer is a Family Problem

The challenges of coping with cancer reverberate through the patient's extended family. Stress on family members may be as great or greater than that experienced by the patient, and increasing emotional pressures can put a tremendous strain on close relationships (Given *et al.* 1993; McCorkle *et al.* 1993; Gilbar *et al.* 1995; Harrison *et al.* 1995; Northouse 1995). So vital to the care of cancer patients is an understanding of the needs of their families that three recent books have been written on the subject, two of which focus on communication: *Cancer and the Family* (Baider *et al.* 1996), *Relating to the Relatives: Breaking Bad News, Communication and Support* (Brewin and Sparshott 1996) and *Talking to Cancer Patients and their Relatives* (Faulkner and Maguire 1996).

Cancer affects the family in a number of ways, the most obvious being the shared crisis. This usually manifests itself as increased symptoms of anxiety, irritability or depression. Families often get locked into the strongly held belief that the healthy partner must not show how upset he or she is because it will add to the worries of the patient. Emotions get bottled up and problems remain unresolved. This can, of course, also happen in reverse, with patients suppressing feelings because they do not wish to worry their families.

Family Members' Reactions to a Loved One's Cancer

Partners may express a gamut of emotions on learning the diagnosis (Euster 1984), and helpers should be prepared for strong emotional reactions. Family members must cope with the patient's emotional reaction to diagnosis and treatment, and with real physical changes in their loved one. Fears about death and the impact on young children may predominate in a partner's mind, who may or may not be able to express these feelings openly. There may be worries about the effect of the cancer on sexual intimacy, although this will depend on the type of cancer and the degree of impact on sexual functioning (Chapter 5). Children often fear that their parent will die, while the adult patient tends to worry about the future of the children when they die.

In the hospital admission interview, it is important to ascertain who is the 'most significant other' for the patient (Gates 1988). The most significant other may be a partner, but it may also be a parent, child, sibling, lover, friend, neighbour or employer. The supportive process is the same. Among the aged, the most significant other may not be a relative. A priest, psychotherapist or volunteer worker may be a most significant other to certain patients. Single, socially isolated, unsupported patients are at particular risk. Assumptions should not be made about the support system until the patient is asked, 'Who is the person closest to you?' or 'Who do you usually turn to when you have problems?'

Once it has been ascertained who is the most significant other, the following questions may help to clarify the nature of support provided by this person (Gates 1988):

What is your history together?

Have you had serious discord?

Have you been estranged?

Have you had counselling? If so, what were the issues and have they been resolved?

Have you ever faced a similar stress? If so, how did you manage?

What is your pattern on the traditional conflicts over money, sex, raising children, religion, politics, etc.?

How does each of you go about being difficult?

How are your differences resolved?

Patients at increased risk of psychological problems tend to have less stable family relationships, lack emotional support, have suffered a recent loss, carry a heavy burden of troubles themselves or have a most significant other with a heavy burden of such problems. It is not possible to know about social problems in the patient without enquiring about them. Divorced and separated people may not wish the estranged party to know they are ill or dying. A lover may be a most significant other. Although progress has been made since the advent of AIDS, many staff are embarrassed to ask about the most significant other in homosexual couples and are still less likely to enquire into the quality of that relationship. Real opportunities for helping are missed in the process.

The family is likely to have been affected by stories of relatives and friends who have died horribly of cancer. Stigma may be important and superstitious beliefs are commonplace. Fears of contagion still persist among many people and some families become isolated by their affliction. Cancer remains a taboo subject for many. Future plans are thwarted and worries set in: 'Will she suffer?' 'How much of a burden will she become?' 'How will it affect the children?' 'Will we be able to withstand the strain?' 'Will she do better if she is left alone, or would she do better to talk about it to us?' (Maguire 1980).

Surgery may leave a patient feeling mutilated and sexually unattractive, prompting fears of rejection by a partner; this can be compounded by the loss of libido that typically follows radiotherapy. The side effects of radiotherapy or chemotherapy treatments may follow, and provision of a wig may do little to allay the trauma of hair loss. Families may question the wisdom of continuing adjuvant therapies in the face of such suffering. Some families become unsympathetic and tell the patient to 'pull yourself together'. Patients may begin to experience feelings of shame that they cannot cope as well as they used to. They may begin to feel fed up with their families.

Partners of cancer patients can suffer a range of psycho-somatic and emotional problems: sleep disturbance, loss of appetite, concentration problems, headaches, worry and fatigue. During the diagnostic phase, shock, uncertainy and a tremendous release of emotions can occur, often followed by exhaustion. In the recurrent phase, fear and anger may predominate because of the return of the disease. In the terminal phase, the principal feelings may be despair, isolation, loneliness, helplessness and loss as partners watch their loved one suffer. Watching the patient in pain and not knowing how to alleviate the suffering is a major problem for families. There is also the possibility of a feeling of isolation among family members when the patient is getting all the attention. As one partner said (Northouse 1988), 'Nobody understands what I'm going through. He's feeling better and I keep feeling worse. Everyone pats him on the back and says how well he's managing. No one asks about me.' Partners' reactions are explored further in Chapter 5.

Problems may arise around care-giving at home. There may be fears of leaving an ill parent alone. Sometimes there is no one whom the family could call on to stay with a patient. Carers may fear they are not doing enough or could cause a mishap. Many relatives experience fears of being inadequate to the task. Also care-givers, like patients, are frequently older with their own health problems.

Difference in Coping Style between Patients and their Partners

Sometimes there are substantial differences between the patient's and the partner's psychological reactions that prevent them from acknowledging feelings, as illustrated in the case of Mrs S.

> Mrs S was diagnosed with an incurable cancer of the lung. She coped with her fears of dying by completely avoiding thinking or talking about them or the seriousness of the illness. Following treatment, the disease was stable but not cured, and she was discharged home. She heard only from the doctor those reassuring words that the disease 'was stable', and in conversation with her husband she referred to future plans and things she would do

continued

continued

> when she got better. The husband, however, was deeply saddened
> and grieved for the wife he was going to lose in the not too
> distant future. He worried about their young children and about
> financial problems that had arisen as a result of the illness. His
> worry was all the more intolerable because of his wife's psycho-
> logical defences, which precluded acknowledging the seriousness
> of the illness and prevented them from sharing feelings in any real
> way.

These differences in psychological reaction and coping style are not uncommon and can contribute to discord between couples and to a breakdown in family relationships. More often than not they add to the strain being placed upon the patient.

The Conspiracy of Silence

Sometimes the family invokes a conspiracy of silence, an insistence by the partner or parents that the patient should not be told of the extent of disease or the prognosis. In some instances, although increasingly rare, they may insist that the patient should not be told the diagnosis *is* cancer. This is done for what the family consider to be good reasons – to help to maintain the patient's morale and hope. Where they insist upon this, any tacit agreement by staff to join the subterfuge usually leads to the situation where it becomes necessary to lie to the patient or be evasive. However, *sometimes the withholding of information can have benefits for the patient and should not be dismissed as always wrong*. Where patients themselves indicate by one means or another that they do not want to be told all, it is entirely appropriate not to give details. The problem for families arises where there is a mismatch between how much the patient wants to know and how much the partner wants to know. For one of them to be privy to information not shared by the other is an isolating experience and carries an emotional cost because family members cannot talk about worries they are not supposed to have. Clearly, each situation needs to be considered individually and with flexibility.

The conspiracy of silence is based on the premise that the patient will not learn the diagnosis or prognosis unless he or she is explicitly told. This is a dangerous assumption. In reality, people usually discover that something is seriously wrong, and it is often impossible for those around the patient to hide everything all the time. The emotions of the family and sometimes of the medical and nursing staff, may be expressed unconsciously or unwittingly through their behaviour. More obviously, where physical symptoms increase and cause limitations and problems for patients, they may interpret these as a sign that they are indeed quite ill. If they are not getting better and feel increasingly ill, the idea that their health is fine becomes untenable. This conspiracy of silence may, therefore, cause more problems than it solves, because of the previous failure to disclose information and the fact that it creates a barrier between family member and patient.

Families at Risk

When there is a poor prognosis for the patient, when the family has difficulties dealing with the cancer and when there are other stressors and limited family coping resources, there is greater risk of psychological problems (Northouse 1995). Several researchers have identified types of family at risk. Weihs and Reiss (1996) base their analysis on the family's security of attachment. Cancer poses the risk of separations and losses that are best dealt with in family relationships that are secure. Families with insecure attachment will be most at risk for prolonged distress. Insecurely attached families come in at least three forms: **ambivalent/preoccupied, avoiding/ dismissing** and **disorganized**. All three will experience difficulties in care-giving, communication, joint problem-solving and capacity for change.

Kissane *et al.* (1994) propose a somewhat different and probably overlapping classification based on the dimensions of cohesion, emotional expressiveness and conflict. **Supportive** families are intimate with each other and share their distress. They are least likely to develop psychological problems, and staff tend to enjoy working with them. At the most severe end of the continuum are **hostile** families, who engage in conflict, find fault, blame, promote guilt and refuse to speak to other members. Their distress reverberates through the treatment system. Somewhat less dysfunctional but nevertheless difficult are **sullen** families, who show a moderate level of conflict and tend to have poor cohesion and emotional expressiveness. Such a classification may assist counsellors in assessing family resilience at the time of diagnosis or terminal illness.

Family therapists are accustomed to working with **enmeshed** families who are at one end of the cohesion continuum while **disengaged** families are at the other (Schulz *et al.* 1996). In enmeshed families, boundaries between people and generations are not observed, people 'live in one another's pockets' and there are few private areas, physical or psychological. Individual family members may be symbiotically enmeshed with another. When one of this symbiotic pair develops cancer, a crisis ensues. In disengaged families, people lead separate lives under one roof and are emotionally disconnected. When a member of such a family falls ill, there may be little or no support coming from relatives. Both types of family can prove difficult to help.

Certain family roles are evident in assessment interviews: for example the **family spokesperson** to whom everyone else defers, the **dominant relative** who takes charge and may engage in bullying tactics with staff to obtain information, the **lonely relative** who is the only one left in the family aside from the patient, and the **outcast** who because of longstanding family feuds is kept from hearing the news of a relative's cancer but may find out in due course (Faulkner and Maguire 1996). All of these individuals can pose communication problems for staff. Another meaning of the family spokesperson may be adaptive – that is, one individual in the family is identified by staff as the person to whom news is given and from whom other family members may hear news about the patient.

Brewin and Sparshott (1996) distinguish between the relative as **advisor and carer**, and the relative as **victim**. Issues to consider in assessing the relative as carer include their psychological state, their theories about the cause of the illness, the quality of their relationship with the patient and whether they and the patient tend to cope with stress in different ways. In assessing the relative as victim, it is important to enquire about previous major stresses or crises, serious past illnesses, both mental and physical, and the presence of a confidante to turn to for support.

Children's Reactions to a Parent's Cancer

Relationships between parents and children bring special problems. There is a set of complicated issues when the child is the patient, and these have been thoroughly reviewed elsewhere (Lansdown and Goldman 1991; van Veldhuisen and Last 1991). Many of the problems surrounding truth-telling with adults are similar for children. Where the parent is the patient, the communication difficulty tends to relate specifically to the issue of what to tell the children, especially when they are not mature enough to fully understand. The desire is often to protect children and prevent them from becoming unnecessarily distressed. Therefore, preadolescent children may be excluded from events to a certain extent. They may not be taken on hospital visits if the patient is unwell or if there is a lot of strange medical equipment around the bed. More often than not this strategy involves not telling the whole truth. A recent study suggests that children are more vulnerable psychologically during a parent's terminal phase of illness than immediately after the loss (Siegel *et al.* 1996a).

What children are told will be limited by their maturity and their ability to understand (Rittenberg 1996). For young children the fantasy may be worse than the reality (Lansdown and Goldman 1988). Explanations given in a way that the child can understand and from the security and support of the family may well be preferable to constructing an elaborate fabrication. If all is not well, even very young children will often pick this up. The danger of lying in this situation is that trust is lost and a lot of hard work is necessary to regain it. One recent study suggests that the most anxious children are those who are unable, for whatever reason, to discuss the parent's illness with their parents (Nelson *et al.* 1994). More than anything else children, like adults, need to be able to anticipate and prepare for what is just around the corner. The issue about what to tell the young children of adults with cancer needs to be carefully addressed and a flexible approach is needed. An important guideline is to listen carefully to what the child is asking – he or she will often come at it obliquely rather than ask straight out – and to reply as clearly and truthfully as possible. As Lansdown and Goldman (1988) suggest, 'the closer to the truth the better'.

Withholding information from children is often rationalized as protecting them from things they are not yet old enough to understand. However, ill parents may fear breaking down in front of their child, experience guilt over abandoning them or feel intense grief over the loss of the opportunity to see them grow up. Ill parents who withhold information are frequently protecting themselves from distress as much as their children. This defence can develop even in well-functioning families. Some children of cancer patients have reported that while they were aware of their parent's illness, they had been given no advance warning of their death and, therefore, had no opportunity to prepare for the loss or say goodbye (Siegel *et al.* 1996b).

Children of ill parents may have difficulties at school, experience sleep and eating disturbances, show increased aggression, have trouble relating to peers and exhibit antisocial behaviour such as stealing. Between the ages of 7 and 10, sadness, worry and loneliness, concern about the safety of the family and worry whether the cancer will return tend to predominate. In children between 10 and 13, the focus is often on the disruption and change a parent's cancer has on their lives. Adolescent children may feel torn between wanting to be with the ill parent but also wishing to separate and do their own thing. Acting-out behaviour is not uncommon among adolescents.

Young children may take a morbid interest in what has happened to an amputated body part or make jokes about a breast prosthesis, playing with it as if it were a toy, throwing it about the room, even giving it a pet name. Young mothers can be helped to deal with these problems in advance through sensitive counselling by hospital staff. 'How do you think you will cope when your little boy discovers that you've lost a breast?' is a good opening question for this kind of discussion.

Among daughters of mastectomy patients, the relationship may be complicated by fears of inheriting breast cancer, rivalry between mother and daughter and the high degree of support some mothers expect from daughters as opposed to sons (Wellisch *et al.* 1992). There are a number of questions that are useful for those counselling distressed adult daughters of breast cancer patients (Wellisch *et al.* 1996).

> Has the mother's illness or death led the daughter to avoid intimate relationships out of a fear of transmitting the suspected gene to her own children?
>
> Does the daughter whose mother developed the disease when she was developing sexually now have guilt or conflicts over her sexuality?
>
> Did a daughter whose mother died have a father who was pathologically dependent or seductive, complicating the daughter's emotional recovery? Or did he remarry quickly, pushing out the memory of mother?
>
> Is there unresolved, internalized anger in the daughter that has crystallized into chronic subclinical depression?
>
> Was the mother an anxious denier who postponed having treatment and used the same coping strategy in dealing with her death, thus preventing discussion with her daughter? Has this style been internalized by the daughter?
>
> Did the mother need to appear as 'superwoman', so that neither mother nor daughter can express negative feelings?

Cultural Variations in Family Response

All ethnic groups are heterogeneous despite prevailing stereotypes, and each family needs to be met individually. At another level, however, some helpful generalizations can be made. Gotay (1996) has identified a number of differences between Anglo and Asian families when a family member has cancer. The terror provoked by the word 'cancer' may be greater in Asian than Anglo families, but it is more likely that Asian family members will wish to protect the patient from unwelcome news than is the case in Anglo families. Some cultures hold a different view of medicine and illness; for example Eastern medicine often explains illness in terms of internal disharmony. In some ethnic groups, coping is family-focused rather than individualized; in Anglo families, death is something to be 'beaten' whereas in some cultures it is accepted as a natural part of the life cycle.

Counsellor sensitivity to cultural beliefs and practices is important, including the role of women in the family, attitudes toward psychosexual problems, faith healing and belief in the role of malign spiritual forces in illness, the importance of the extended family, and rituals at the time of death. Common difficulties in detecting psychological distress in patients of ethnic minorities include varying expressions of distress, inhibition of cues of depression from the patient, difficulties in judging the patient's demeanour, ascribing abnormal behaviour to cultural factors and misinterpreting culturally appropriate behaviour (Patel 1996).

For many ethnic groups, to be seen suffering brings shame to the family, including previous generations. Highly valued among Asian and some Afro-Caribbean communities are women who are 'copers', sacrificing their own needs to protect the family's honour. Seeking help for emotional problems is viewed negatively; therefore, many of these women who find their way to help are in crisis situations (Dosanjh *et al.* 1977). Some of the coping responses described in Chapter 3 might be considered appropriate in one culture but pathological in another. As helpers we must always try to be aware of how our own cultural stereotypes influence our interpretation of patients' responses to cancer and to remember that the needs of families in different ethnic groups may vary tremendously.

Staff Relationships with Family Members

Typically, contacts between health professionals and family members are limited. Families tend to visit patients in hospital in the afternoons and evenings, while ward rounds are often in the morning. Family members usually have to take the initiative to talk to the doctor, and they are often hesitant to 'bother' staff. Professionals tend not to initiate interactions with carers unless there is a change in the patient's condition. Family members have a high need for information about the patient and often view health professionals as controllers of that information. It is helpful when staff try to anticipate family members' needs (Northouse 1988).

It is clear that, when family dynamics are positive and healthy, people with cancer can derive immense benefit from the support of those who love them. Bluglass (1991) argues for the importance of the health care team in developing a relationship with patients' families, not only to aid coping but also to gain their support in facilitating treatment compliance and management. Indeed Rait and Lederberg (1989) urge all professionals working in this area to 'think family', and Northouse (1995) urges clinicians to make family-based assessments rather than narrower patient-based assessments. Research highlights the risk of increased psychological difficulty if social and family support is lacking (Gilbar *et al.* 1995). In a health care system primarily oriented to the patient, it is easy to forget that effective communication skills demand a family orientation. It is simply not possible to work effectively with patients and ignore the fact that somewhere in the background are family members, close friends or partners who have an important influence as care-givers.

5
Couples' Issues and Psychosexual Problems

The Impact of Cancer on the Couple

Cancer brings some couples closer together, but other relationships are at risk of experiencing a crisis. Peteet and Greenberg (1995) describe four types of couple who are at particular risk. In an **immature** relationship, commitment has not been tested, partners are unaccustomed to relying on one another and the relationship enters a crisis when one partner tries to lean on an unempathic partner. The counsellor may need to suggest time apart from one another and respect for the other's coping style. The needier partner may require extra support. Cancer may contribute to the dissolution of some immature relationships if it discloses major differences between the partners. In **hostile–dependent** relationships, partners are enmeshed in a relationship marked by a high degree of conflict and distorted communication. Threats to leave or volatile arguments may alternate with uneasy periods of calm. These couples are helped to find an area of consensus in order to improve communication. They may require couples therapy.

Occasionally oncology staff will learn of an episode of the physical abuse of a patient by a partner, which puts the patient medically and psychologically at risk. **Physically abusive** relationships require monitoring in order to promote safety for patient and family. In **estranged** relationships, characterized by emotional detachment, cancer can provoke a crisis when the patient realizes the lack of intimacy and emotional relatedness in the relationship. Such patients may seriously consider leaving a partner, which may pose additional problems. In such cases, counsellors can help by clarifying the areas of disappointment and exploring what support is available in the relationship. Features of more than one of these four types may be present in a single relationship.

Cancer patients without partners should not be forgotten. Many of these patients – single, widowed, separated or divorced – are at high risk for depression if they lack a network of support. Young, never-married cancer patients may have deep concerns about whether they will be attractive to a partner, be able to perform sexually or become parents. When the quality of a marital or cohabiting relationship is good, having a partner is associated with less distress, but patients in poorly functioning relationships have more problems (Rodrigue and Park 1996). Good communication in the partner relationship is characterized by high levels of empathy and a low incidence of emotional withdrawal (Pistrang and Barker 1995). Distress is greatly elevated among partners of terminally ill cancer patients (Siegel *et al.* 1996c).

Psychosexual Issues in Cancer

One aspect of working with the partners of cancer patients deserves special attention and that is the range of sexual side effects of the illness, surgery and treatment. Throughout treatment, sexual consequences should be considered and discussed with the patient. The patient's sexual partner should be included in consultations whenever possible, and touching and sex should be discussed along with other aspects of recuperation. Patients may need to be encouraged to be physically affectionate with their partners and to return gradually to sexual activity (Zilbergeld 1979).

An assessment of the likelihood of sexual dysfunction includes the following factors (Schain 1981):

- the meaning to the patient of cancer and of the particular body part involved

- the degree of visibility of organ alteration and the stigma associated with that change

- the impact of treatments on self-esteem and on sexual/ hormonal functioning

- pretreatment sexual attitudes, personality profile and favoured coping strategies

- social support, life stage at the time of diagnosis, former adaptation to stress

- whether the disease is likely to have a catastrophic or consolidating effect on the patient's defences and self-esteem.

At least four sexual problem areas typically arise in cancer treatment:

- the alteration in body image as a result of the disease, surgery or treatment

- the inability to have sexual intercourse, usually as a result of surgery, chemotherapy, radiotherapy or hormone therapy

- infertility secondary to cancer therapy or surgery

- fears of abandonment by one's partner.

Alternative forms of sexual activity may need to be discussed: masturbation or mutual masturbation, mutual arousal techniques such as caressing, fondling and kissing, oral-genital stimulation, artificial aids such as vibrators and coital alternatives such as oral-genital sex.

Helpers who feel uncomfortable or unconfident in raising these issues might need to consider referral of the patient and partner to a specialist counsellor or sex therapist. Recent technical developments have enhanced sexual performance for some patients and addressed infertility issues: breast reconstruction, vaginal reconstruction, penile implants, ova saving, IVF, sperm banking, artificial insemination and hormone therapies aimed at correcting the imbalance caused by disruption to gonadal function (Fisher 1983; Ostroff and Lesko 1991).

The impacts of cancer on body image are many: surgery that leaves a scar or removes a body part, the creation of an artificial opening in the abdominal wall fitted with a bag to collect faeces (in colostomy), the use of indwelling catheters to collect urine, radiation effects, chemotherapy effects and the effects of hormonal therapy. Treatments for cancer may have a profound effect on all phases of the sexual response: sexual desire and interest, arousal, congestion of the genitals and orgasm. The loss of genital parts is the most obvious cause of dysfunction: removal of the breast and 'catastrophic' surgery for genital maligancies, such as excision of the vulva and clearance of the abdominal cavity in women and amputation of the testicles or penis in men. However the impact on sexual function of chronic pain and of anxiety and depression must also be considered, and disruption in sexual activity by chemotherapy is very common.

What can health care staff do? They can detail the effects on sexual response of treatments the patient is undergoing, explain the diagnostic tests available to find the cause of a sexual problem, describe ways to cope with appliances during sexual activity, suggest methods that compensate for inadequate vaginal lubrication, minimize painful intercourse or help the resumption of sex comfortably after an illness and encourage couples to continue noncoital caressing to orgasm when intercourse is not possible (Schover 1986).

Patients undergoing radical surgery for pelvic or genital cancer have special needs. The preoperative assessment of sexual functioning should be careful and detailed. Starting with the least sensitive material, the couple are invited to talk about their relationship generally. Simple language can be used to describe the genitals and different kinds of sexual activity. Open-ended questions elicit the most information, for example, 'How do you feel about oral sex?' rather than 'Have you tried oral sex?' Normalizing language can help a patient feel comfortable about revealing sexual material. For example, 'I've noticed that many husbands worry that their wives might catch bladder cancer through sexual intercourse. What

thoughts do you have about that?' When surgery is likely to
disrupt sexual function, a clear preoperative explanation using
an anatomical model can be of great benefit to the patient
(Schover and Fife 1985).

Auchincloss (1989) has usefully listed the type and extent of
psychosexual problems likely to be experienced by patients
with different kinds of cancer (Table 5.1) (Auchincloss 1989).

Table 5.1 Psychosexual problems associated with different cancers
(Auchincloss 1989)

Site of cancer	Psychosexual issues
Breast	Significance of the breast, emotional and sexual appearance concerns – scar, prosthesis, reconstruction, surgical treatment – loss of breast Chemotherapy: loss of ovarian function Young patients: fertility after treatment
Gynaecological sites	Significance of female genital organs (emotional, sexual, reproductive) Surgical treatment: loss of uterus, ovaries, vagina or external genitalia Chemotherapy: loss of ovarian function Appearance concerns Radiation therapy: fibrosis and scarring of the vagina Sexual dysfunction: fear of pain with intercourse, other concerns, loss of childbearing capacity
Testicular sites	Significance of testes (emotional, sexual, reproductive) Appearance concerns: prosthesis Chemotherapy: sterility or changes in ejaculation Surgery: sterility or changes in ejaculation Sperm banking
Bladder, prostate, colon, rectum	High incidence of impotence after surgery Impact of colostomy, even when temporary
Lymphoma, leukaemia	Long, stressful treatment Appearance concerns Chemotherapy: can cause sterility, loss of ovarian function

However other cancers also deserve attention, such as disfiguring facial surgery in head and neck cancers, lung cancer (the commonest site of cancer) and sarcomas requiring limb amputation. Those undergoing genital surgery are not the only cancer patients with sexual problems. In the case of amputees, reactions vary from depressive withdrawal and passivity to angry refusal to accept any limitations. It is vital to include partners in rehabilitation. Phantom limb pain should be enquired about and treated effectively. Phantom breast and phantom rectum may occur after surgery and may need to be discussed. The patient has a need to grieve for what is lost as a result of the amputation, especially if there was little time to prepare for the loss (Parkes 1982). Doing a sexual assessment is also important to ascertain the level of psychosexual dysfunction before cancer treatment. Research with bone marrow transplant patients found very high levels of psychosexual dysfunction prior to initiation of chemotherapy (Marks *et al.* 1996).

There are a number of common staff attitudes or myths that lead to the avoidance of sexual issues with cancer patients: 'It's not my job.' 'It takes special training.' 'It takes a lot of time.' 'Sex therapy is only for healthy people.' 'There isn't any treatment, so it's cruel to even bring it up.' 'He or she should be grateful to be alive.' 'What if he or she falls apart when I ask?' 'I'm too uncomfortable talking about sex.' 'I would bring it up if this patient were married.' 'I might bring it up if this patient were younger.' 'I should bring it up, but I think this patient is gay.' 'If it's a real problem, he or she'll mention it.' 'It'll probably take care of itself with time.' 'If he or she brings it up again, I'll do something about it' (Auchincloss 1989). Patients do not usually mention these issues spontaneously and there is significant under-reporting of problems. Once asked, people will often offer information freely about their sexual difficulties.

Learning to ask about sexual health is part of health care staff's responsibility. As with other difficult questions, there is a tendency to assume that someone else is attending to this aspect of the patient's needs. Contrary to the myths listed above, most cancer patients have sexual concerns. It must not be assumed that older patients have no interest in sex. Single patients of any age often doubt that anyone will ever find them desirable again. 'And how are things on the sexual side?' should be a routine part of every follow-up. More detailed invitations to say more about the sexual side include comments such as these:

> Sometimes during this treatment, people find they have lost interest in lovemaking.
>
> People sometimes worry about how their partners will respond to them sexually after this operation.
>
> Some people find it difficult to resume their usual pattern of lovemaking after surgery.
>
> Some women are very distressed about their change in shape.
>
> Some people worry that their partner might reject them after this operation.

Special problems arise with people with AIDS. When the patient has acquired the disease from a partner, the able-bodied lover is often left feeling, 'I killed the person I love through the act of loving'. In these circumstances, great sensitivity and skill are required to deal with the range of feelings in the patient, the partner, their families and friends.

Taking a sexual history is best done at or soon after diagnosis. This conveys to the patient that sex is an appropriate topic to bring up at future visits. The briefest sexual history should include current sexual status, current relationships and past sexual history. With more time, family background, attitudes toward sex, and cancer myths relating to sexual function can be covered. The nonverbal stance to take is important and requires that the helper is comfortable enough with sexual matters to speak about them openly and without embarrassment to patients of any age. This is probably an area in which many staff would welcome a postqualification study day, but it should be covered as a topic in basic medical and nursing training.

The simple fact of asking about sexual function is reassuring to patients. It conveys that the topic is acceptable, that concerns can freely be raised and that problems which arise later can be discussed and treated. The following is an example of a blunder that could have been avoided by asking the appropriate question preoperatively (Auchincloss 1989):

A woman was reassured after vulvectomy [removal of the vulva] that she would be able to have comfortable intercourse. However, it was unknown to her physician (who never asked) that she was homosexual and had enjoyed clitoral stimulation rather than intercourse with her partner of many years. In treatment it came out that she was able to reach orgasm with intravaginal stimulation alone, which contributed to a good outcome.

Some health professionals are wary of discussing sexual matters with patients because of limited knowledge. The PLISSIT model is a simple intervention that can be made by those without specialized training in sex therapy:

P   permission to be sexual while ill or undergoing treatment

LI   limited information

SS   specific suggestion (for example, alternatives to intercourse, position changes to decrease discomfort)

IT   intensive therapy, when deeper underlying problems are present.

In general, 70% of patients respond to the first three levels (PLISS). For the remaining 30%, giving a referral to a qualified colleague may be one of the helper's most important functions (Shipes and Lehr 1982).

The psychosexual problems of patients undergoing colostomy and mastectomy are especially challenging and deserve separate consideration. Specialist stoma and mastectomy nurses are now on the staff of most general hospitals, but other health professionals who come in contact with these patients need to be aware of the sensitive psychological issues involved.

Psychosexual Aspects of Colostomy

'The sight of one's gut sticking out spewing forth faeces' (Dlin 1973) is not an easy matter for most people. Orbach *et al.* (1957) reported the emotional reactions of people who had recently undergone this operation. Like other first-person accounts in this book, they are included in order to give the helper some idea of the patient's experience, because until helpers have allowed the experience of cancer to have an emotional impact on them, they will probably be poorly prepared to help.

> *I had a spillage once from eating a pear shortly after the operation when I first came home from the hospital. I was at home when it happened and it spilled all over the floor and myself because I was unable to get to the bathroom in time. This is something you never forget.*

> *It happened outside of my home about a year ago. I was in the store when it went 'bang, gush' and it spilled all over me. I felt so panicky that I didn't dare to take a cab but ran through the streets hoping and praying that no one would stop to speak to me.*

Patients who have had surgery for colorectal cancer have high levels of physical, psychological, social and sexual dysfunction (Sprangers *et al.* 1993). There are the practical problems of handling the stoma: irrigation, changing bags and leakage. There is often impaired self-esteem and psychological dysfunction, with depression and anxiety. Anxiety in social situations and fears of sexual undesirability are widespread. Often there is either impaired sexual function or fears about sex when sexual function is actually unimpaired. The operation and its aftermath place a strain on key personal and work relationships, and social isolation can result (Hurny and Holland 1985). Gloeckner (1983) describes how patients sometimes wait a year or more before showing the stoma to a partner. First sexual experiences following surgery may be overwhelmingly warm and affirming or result in a feeling of rejection. Accidents with appliances during love-making can cause considerable strain. It is also well to remember the following observation (Hurny and Holland 1985).

> *Orgasm can be experienced without erection and ejaculation. It is a psycho-physiological experience of the individual, possible even after penectomy [removal of the penis]. Many of the patients we studied with bladder and colon cancer were able to experience orgasm through oral stimulation, for example, without erection or ejaculation. Inability to have an erection after pelvic surgery can [also] be reversed by surgical implantation of a prosthesis.*

However, the loss of sexual potency is a serious matter and when surgery carries with it a high incidence of this complication, the surgeon should discuss this possibility with the patient (Bernstein 1972):

> *A few years ago I performed an abdominoperineal resection [surgery for cancer of the colon] on a male patient, aged 83. I failed to discuss the probability of sexual impotence with him. About four months after the operation I was somewhat surprised to have the patient put the following question to me: 'Doctor, when can I expect my manhood to return?'*

Some surgeons are reluctant to mention the possibility of impotence preoperatively because they fear they will plant in the patient's mind the seeds of the very complication they hope to avoid (Burton and Parker 1997).

Patients with an **ileal conduit** for malignant disease in association with the bladder should also be discussed here. Urine is collected in a drainable appliance, requiring four to six drainages a day. Like other stomas, the conduit is prone to leakage, sore skin, odour and surgical complications. Psychological outcome for these patients resembles that of other patients with stomas. Change in body image and sexual dysfunction can occur. To improve sexual adjustment, nightshirts, camisoles and crotchless underpants can be used to conceal the appliance (Bourke 1984).

The creation of an artificial opening in the abdomen is a procedure of last resort to save a life. The operation creates an unnatural state of affairs that causes considerable stress at both conscious and unconscious levels. All of the body openings are invested with emotional energy and meaning and, in the anthropological sense, may be considered potentially dangerous. In assessing the likelihood of complications, Dlin (1973) enumerates factors to explore before the operation:

> *How resilient is the patient under stress?*
> *What is the symbolic meaning of the operation to the patient – what does 'closing an opening' and 'opening a closing' conjure up in the patient's mind?*
> *Is there a wish to live or a wish to die?*

Unconscious wishes to die are not uncommon in cancer patients. Surgery may be seen as a way out of problems, with the surgeon or anaesthetist as executioner. Special attention needs to be paid in this regard to Engel's (1968) 'giving up–given up complex'. This is an attitude characterized by helplessness or hopelessness, low self-image, loss of gratification from relationships or roles in life, a disruption of continuity between past, present and future, and a reactivation under stress of memories of earlier periods of giving up. Apathy is a particularly ominous preoperative danger sign for colostomy or for any cancer surgery.

After a colostomy, toilet training must begin again and long-repressed conflicts that were faced around the age of two must be resolved a second time (Dlin 1973). Helpers need to be sensitive to the fact that the psychological issues of the second year of life must be renegotiated by the patient. 'The twin stigmata of faeces and cancer, coupled with the shame and embarrassment of stoma life' may cause formidable problems for individual patients (Fallowfield and Clark 1994). Potential problems include management of appliances, reaction to spillage, mourning the lost body part, and possibly phantom rectum (just as mastectomy patients sometimes experience phantom breast). Homosexual men may experience considerable problems following surgery that removes the anus and rectum, in which case alternatives to penetrative anal sex can be explored and discussed.

The unconscious meaning of the stoma may be important. The stoma is sometimes seen as a phallus, especially by women, who occasionally call it their 'little peter'. Areas of the body where skin and mucous membranes meet have special properties: they are on the surface, they can be manipulated and rhythmic repeated stimulation leads to a tension and satisfaction cycle. However such thoughts and feelings may be difficult for patients to put into words (Dlin 1973).

Ways of concealing the appliance during lovemaking may need to be discussed. Some female patients conceal the bag underneath a sexy pair of knickers. Sometimes, postoperative impotence occurs in men that is psychological rather than physiological and origin, and in-depth counselling can help to restore their potency. On average, it takes about a year to adjust to living with a stoma. A number of substantial difficulties need to be negotiated, and allowances need to be made for slow progress in some cases (Dlin 1973).

Psychosexual Aspects of Mastectomy

Sexual problems are very common after mastectomy. One study found that after mastectomy 44% of women experienced a general decrease in sexual activity, 39% wore less revealing night clothes, 36% did not undress completely in front of their partner, 36% had intercourse with a bra or top on, 28% engaged in less foreplay and initiated sex play less often and 26% had sexual relations with the lights out (Abt *et al.* 1978).

Self-conscious about the prosthesis, some women fail to return to work although they are well enough to do so. Very anxious women may examine their breasts up to 60 times a day and consult their doctor regularly. Behaviour such as this can tax partners' patience to breaking point. In one study of the partners of mastectomy patients, few discussed their worries with anyone. Most felt they had not been allowed to play a sufficient part in the decision-making about the operation, some were very anxious or depressed, sexual problems were common, some had difficulties in their work and some said their social life had diminished. Others felt the illness and surgery had brought them closer to their partners (Maguire 1980).

If a patient refuses to allow her partner to be present for discussions prior to surgery, or if the partner declines to attend, the possibility of difficulties within the couple should be raised. It is helpful to inform the partner that the patient may be very worried about her health and this is understandable. A good deal of courage may be required for a woman to let her partner see the scar, and she may watch carefully for signs of rejection. Some mothers find it very difficult to discuss the operation with daughters or to show them the scar. Some mothers with older sons feel diminished by the operation and fear their sons will no longer find them acceptable. In the case of younger children, mothers are often more uncertain about letting little ones know what has happened. They may concoct cover stories or refuse to cuddle them in case the child should notice they have lost a breast. Some mothers ensure that their children cannot see them naked (Maguire 1980).

In 1955, Bard and Sutherland described the emotional impact

of breast cancer and mastectomy on women. This remains one of the finest early studies of the emotional impact of cancer on patients.

> *I can't look at it ... I haven't cried like this before in my life. But I can't help it. I know there is nothing that can be done ... They told me they were going to take it out, but they took the whole thing off. I never would have let them. I'm even ashamed to walk down the street. I'm ashamed to let them see me in the neighbourhood. I think everybody is looking at me.*

Patients described vivid preoperative dreams:

> *I was walking down the gangplank of a ferry boat with a lot of other women. At the bottom of the gangplank was a man and he was checking each woman to see if she had her breasts. I was getting closer to the bottom when I woke up.*

Women who are likely to have special needs after mastectomy are (Schain 1988):

- young and/or single and have a high emotional investment in their breasts
- have not had the number of children they had hoped for, or consider having children to be a major life goal
- may have been sexually abused
- did not get the treatment of their choice
- have few areas of gratification or self-esteem other than their primary relationship
- have a history of substance misuse and/or psychological problems
- have had radiotherapy or chemotherapy.

Other surgery to the breast, either lumpectomy or reconstructive surgery, may also cause problems. It should not be assumed that more conservative surgical procedures will eliminate the sexual problems known to be associated with the loss of the breast. Breast-cancer treatments also carry sexual side effects (Kaplan 1992). Women who are fatigued, have lost their hair and gained weight do not feel sexually desirable, especially when chemotherapy follows mastectomy. Some chemotherapy agents impair fertility and menstruation, and lower sexual desire by interfering with the production of sex hormones. Oestrogen deficiency impairs the female excitement phase, and a premature menopause may also involve androgen deficiency, which impairs sexual desire. Some women taking tamoxifen report soreness, drying and shrinking of the vagina, while others experience a loss of libido and of orgastic response.

6
Communication Problems

Disclosing the Diagnosis and Prognosis

The following statements are representative of complaints women made a year after breast surgery (Burton and Parker 1994).

When they told me [the diagnosis] in outpatients ... I was lying down still naked to the waist ... He asked me if I had any questions. I was bereft of speech. He said he'd answer any questions when I came out. And when I came out, he wasn't there, and sister showed me the way out.

I went to get the results of my biopsy and I was lying on the table half undressed. They were talking about surgery and I got very frightened. 'You don't mean I have cancer, do you?', I asked, and he just said, very offhand, 'Oh yes'.

They never told me for eight days after the operation what they'd found, and it so upset my son. This young doctor breezed in and swept aside the curtains and said, 'It's about time, Mrs. X, you knew you have bowel cancer' [peritoneal secondaries]. I knew there was something serious because they didn't stop at my bed at ward rounds. The registrar just waved his hand towards me and said, 'Oh, tangled bowel, tangled bowel'.

The doctor didn't even take us into the office, he took us into the sluice room on the ward. He said, 'Well, you know we've removed cancer from your breast. There's nothing more we can do. You'll have to take these tablets for the rest of your life. There's no point in coming down to hospital because it'll be a waste of your time. If you find another lump in your breast or under your arm, or if you have pain in your back, or lose weight, go to your own doctor. You could live for five years, you could live for two years, you could live for...' And then he just shrugged his shoulders. Neither my husband nor I has been able to forget that.

In the next passage, a future doctor aged 12 years reflects on the conspiracy of silence surrounding his neuroblastoma (Watts 1993). He had developed pain and weakness in his right leg.

The only information I was given was that I was going to have an operation. My parents were told I had a malignant tumour and there was 'not much expectation of life'. I could tell they were upset.... I soon realised that no one was going to answer questions about the illness.... Once a week the consultant would come round. He would not answer my questions but he did palpate my axillae and groin, then say 'Fine' and then leave. As I knew there was nothing wrong with them, this solitary syllable of reassurance did little for me...

When I was 14 my father caught pulmonary TB and my chest X-ray showed pulmonary opacities. After ineffective treatment for TB, I was admitted for a lobectomy. This time I was treated far better. I was told I had TB, my questions were answered and it made sense until I realised I was the only patient with TB to be given radiotherapy and intravenous injections.... I attended outpatients as a medical student, but still no one would answer relevant questions – even after I had obtained my notes and read them through ... In summary, my illness involved considerable unnecessary stress from feelings of isolation and helplessness.

Why have health professionals avoided giving information to cancer patients? In a 1970s study of doctors on a UK cancer ward, it was found that nearly all believed patients should not be told they had cancer unless it was curable. They assumed patients did not want to know and would react badly to being told. Telling patients the truth would cause them to lose hope. Even a patient who asked outright 'might simply be seeking reassurance' (McIntosh 1978). Patients were fobbed off with euphemisms like 'ulcer' or 'thickening' and when cancer was confirmed, other euphemisms were used such as 'suspicious cells', 'nasty cells', 'activity', or 'something which might have been dangerous'. In the event of life-threatening illness, the word cancer was still not used, but the patient's consent to surgery was obtained through the use of terms such as 'going malignant' or 'would turn cancerous if left alone'. Embodied in these procedures were attempts to limit patients asking further questions.

But of course patients *did* ask further questions, and responses to these were also managed in a routine way. The content of doctors' replies was framed in such a way as to prevent further questions. Patients were told the doctor did not know the diagnosis and further tests would be required. When test results were available, euphemisms were used to conceal the diagnosis. If the patient asked, 'Is it cancer?' the answer was, 'Well, it could certainly have become malignant if it had been left'. If patients refused treatment they were told, 'This could be a danger to your life if it isn't treated'. Despite doctors' stated practice of varying what they told from patient to patient, only in exceptional cases was there a departure from routine. Doctors often used a pretence of uncertainty about the diagnosis, even after the histology report had been received, as a device for avoiding further disclosure: 'suspicious cells' that 'might have become dangerous' (McIntosh 1978).

Since the publication of McIntosh's study, more information about diagnosis and prognosis is now routinely given to cancer patients in the USA and UK (Weil *et al.* 1994; Buckman 1996), but current practices remain widely divergent, especially in Europe and the East. In Norway, 81% of doctors prefer giving the full diagnosis (Loge *et al.* 1996). Gastroenterologists in northern Europe usually reveal the diagnosis to patients and their partners, whereas those in southern and eastern Europe usually conceal the diagnosis from the patient (Thomsen *et al.* 1993). Among surgeons in the Midlands (UK), 45% tell virtually all patients about malignancy while 55% say they are guided by patients' and relatives' wishes; a few say they never tell the patient the diagnosis is cancer, but they always tell relatives (Burton and Parker 1997). Withholding the diagnosis from the patient remains very common in Greece (Mystakidou *et al.* 1996), Spain (Centeno-Cortes and Nunez-Olarte 1994), Italy (Pronzato *et al.* 1994), Singapore (Tan *et al.* 1993) and Taiwan (Ger *et al.* 1996).

There is wide variability from culture to culture in terms of what people with cancer are told. In the USA, the process is controlled by law and an ethos that states that individual responsibility is best and people must take control of their own lives. This contrasts sharply with the oriental view where the individual 'belongs' to the family and decisions and responsibilities are family matters. Where a culture demands individual responsibility, the corollary is the requirement that individuals be fully informed of all that affects their health so that they may take control. USA requirements are inflexible by insisting that explicit discussion of treatment, risks and benefits take place, thus institutionalizing a process that ought to be flexible and individual, and governed first and foremost not by legal requirements but by humane concern for others.

Because of the current trend toward more frank and open disclosure, doctors may find themselves experiencing problems in dealing with the communication of emotionally challenging information to patients and relatives. The paternalism of the medical practitioner has been well-entrenched, and there are many who believe that if the truth is painful then it is better to protect the patient. Recent research suggests that most patients want to know their diagnosis, prognosis, treatment options and possible side effects (Meredith *et al.* 1996). The notion that it is better not to say anything that is upsetting is more widely held than is sometimes obvious. For instance, it is not uncommon to hear other professions complain of the behaviour of mental health colleagues, who when talking to patients have apparently upset them. It is sometimes assumed that this happens because a distressing topic is being raised unnecessarily. This, in fact, is rarely the case. Upset is not usually caused by the process of talking about something, rather talking about it provides an opportunity to disclose existing distress. It is not talking about cancer that is distressing, it is having cancer that is distressing. The mental health professional may feel confident in dealing with the patient's emotions. Others dealing with cancer patients may feel less confident to do so, which may result in limiting emotional expression in patients or relatives.

Patients' dissatisfaction with information given to them by doctors is well documented (Fallowfield *et al.* 1995). Reasons cited for not giving information include time constraints, inadequate training, deliberate withholding of details on the grounds that patients will ask if they want to know, and the knowledge that patients do not retain and may even repress the information given to them, especially if it contains emotionally distressing issues (Hogbin and Fallowfield 1989).

Goldie (1982) points out that the moral issue is not simply whether or not to tell cancer patients the truth, but more importantly how to do so. Lies and the unprepared-for bad news may both be damaging. Putting oneself into the patient's shoes, as doctors often do, is the best way of *not* knowing what another feels, Goldie suggests. There is a danger in assuming that the patient is feeling the way we would be feeling in their shoes, and the helper should always guard against this. This example illuminates the problem (Goldie 1982).

> Mr. P decided, when his cancer of the oesophagus was discovered, to forego any treatment for it. A year later he was referred to the psychotherapist because he was thought to be depressed. When interviewed it turned out that he was depressed because his vision was blurred and he could not coordinate sufficiently to write. And this, it turned out, was due to the side-effects of three drugs which were antidepressants and tranquillisers and three drugs which were for the relief of pain. He had been given these drugs because it was presumed that he would be in pain, yet he said he had never complained of pain. The tranquillisers were given because it was thought he would be anxious as death was close. He said he was not afraid of dying but he was concerned about the possibility of dying through choking, with no relief available. In effect he had been given drugs without having a condition that required them.

Since the advent of surveys of doctors' practices in telling cancer patients their diagnoses, there has been a tendency to identify a doctor either as one who believes that patients should be told the truth or as one who believes they should not. All doctors are supposed to belong to one school or the other, yet most have learned there are important exceptions to every generalization. Brewin (1977) describes five different situations:

- the patient desperately hopes for reassurance that they have not got cancer

- aggressively cheerful optimism: these patients will be deeply upset or angry if they are bluntly given a diagnosis they are striving to reject

- apparently they want 'the full facts', as given to relatives; if the prognosis is bad, further assessment is needed as to what exactly the patient wants to know

- these patients do not want to discuss diagnosis or prognosis; they are often living from day to day, perhaps cheerful, perhaps sad, but reasonably philosophical, confident that everything possible is being done

- tense and suspicious that they are being kept in the dark, some patients badly need more information.

The same phrases that would insult the dignity and intelligence of one patient may bring comfort and encouragement to another: 'having cancer', 'having a curable kind of cancer', 'having a small tumour', or 'having a growth'. Also the same words spoken in the same way by the same doctor can be completely right for one patient and quite wrong for another. Responsiveness to the patient's verbal and nonverbal cues are skills that can be learned (Bennett and Alison 1995).

In the face of the trend toward telling all patients when they have cancer, Brewin and others have put the case for restraint. Slevin (1987) suggests that patients should be given the information they request, but no more initially. Those patients who wish to forget about the illness and leave all decisions to the doctor should be allowed to do so, while those who want to be involved in every aspect of their treatment should be given that opportunity. Whether or not the prognosis and diagnosis are discussed depends on what the patient wants to know. There are clearly some patients who do not want to know the diagnosis at the time of referral, and although they may eventually come to accept the diagnosis after a period of treatment, they may make it very clear that they do not wish to know the outlook. If unwelcome information is given to patients who are using denial or avoidance as a way of coping, many of them will claim to have forgotten it completely: 'I can't remember what he said', one patient said at follow-up. 'Something about lymph. All I know is that I'm under treatment, and *that's all I want to know*' (Burton and Parker 1995).

Problems arise when family members insist the patient must not be told of a cancer before the doctor has had an opportunity to impart the news to the patient. Bennett and Alison (1996) point out that ethically, *clinical information should be discussed with a patient first and with relatives after obtaining the patient's permission* – an ethical principle that is not always known by the lay public. Relatives should be assured that if the patient indicates a clear desire not to be given bad news, this will be respected. A recent study showed that cancer patients wished doctors to respect their views rather than those of their family, should they differ. Almost all patients were opposed to their family influencing the information they would receive about their illness (Benson and Britten 1996).

Special problems arise when patients come from other cultures where the family take decisions about the welfare of ill relatives. Freedman (1993) describes the situation that arose when the Greek–Canadian family of a dying cancer patient insisted she not be told her diagnosis. A decision was required on whether to place a catheter in one of her kidneys because an abdominal mass had obstructed the other kidney. The family threatened to sue at one point when they were told her diagnosis would be revealed. She was asked if she had any questions, and she did not. It was repeated that she was very ill, she was asked if she understood that, and she did. Some patients, it was explained, want to know about their illness – what would she like? She whispered to a relative that she would like to leave it alone for the moment. She delegated treatment decisions to her children, which resolved the situation.

In summary, 'to tell or not to tell' is no longer the issue, but rather what information is appropriate for a particular patient. The full details of diagnosis and prognosis may be as inappropriate as bland reassurance (Hoy 1985).

Breaking Bad News

Often it is the doctor who is at the sharp end of this process, and a substantial literature now exists dealing with this ongoing problem, because bad news does not stop with the diagnosis (Buckman and Kason 1993). Confirming cancer is a piece of bad news; later, when the disease becomes incurable as it disseminates, this is another piece of bad news. Bad news may, however, arise more subtly and more often than is sometimes assumed. Each time the patient has a test or scan, it is possible that the result will be bad news. Each time they are told they will receive more treatment, that can be bad news. So bad news must not be thought of as something that happens at rare critical points but rather as something quite commonplace and frequent.

It is important to avoid assuming that because something is a normal daily phenomenon in medicine, that it is the same for patients. It may be safest to assume that for people with cancer there is threat and challenge in a great deal of the information given. There is a need to listen to what the patient tells us about their response to what they are hearing. When it comes to understanding what patients feel about the information they are given, sometimes we cannot see what we do not look for.

Maguire and Faulkner (1988a) point out that bad news is still bad news whichever way it is given. However, there is clearly a skill to doing this that allows the bearer of bad news to be supportive of the person receiving it. Giving bad news is a two-way process both in communication terms and emotionally. Before deciding at what pace to go and how much to tell, the person disclosing the news needs to be aware of their own motives in this process and the extent to which their own needs may influence the process. Therefore, it is sometimes helpful to ask, 'Why am I doing this in this way, and how far is this dictated by *my* needs and not those of the patient?' As Molleman *et al.* (1984) point out, 'The physician who holds that "patients do not demand much time and attention" and his colleague who holds that "patients demand much time and attention" may ... both see their opinion confirmed by their own behaviour'.

The difficulties of communicating bad news and of doing it well have been eloquently described by Goldberg (1984) and Kelly (1987). Goldberg highlights the doctor's dilemma by drawing attention to the fact that the 'presumed obligation both to inform and to protect can create an ongoing strain for the clinician.... The patient has a need for truth to make decisions. Concealment can undermine trust in the physician and the profession. Further, concealment may be based on physicians' uneasiness rather than patients' inability to accept information.' Kelly (1987) put it more pragmatically and forcefully by saying, '*Information is power*'. With information, people can act as adults to make decisions that are appropriate for them and their lifestyles. Without information, they are more likely to be confused and frightened and will be less prepared to make truly informed decisions.... When people are confused they generally need more information, not less.' The doctor–patient relationship has always been one of unequal power. The patient comes to the doctor for help; the doctor has the power to help with health problems. It is encumbent on doctors, therefore, to be clear about their power and how it is used.

Bad news is any information likely to alter drastically a patient's view of their future, including any alteration to expected lifespan (Buckman 1984). The news that the patient may have cancer, almost certainly has cancer or definitely has cancer all fall into this category. Brewin (1991) describes three ways of giving bad news:

- the blunt and unfeeling way: standing at the foot of the bed in a white coat, looking down at the patient

- the kind and sad way: in private, concerned and unhurried but regarding the matter as just a painful duty

- the understanding and positive way: based on flexibility, feedback, reassurance and planning for the immediate future, all blended with the bad news.

An illustration of the understanding and positive way might be, 'I'm afraid the tests show there is a cancer, but I'm glad to say that the position is at least more hopeful than some cases we see', or 'At least the liver seems normal and healthy, which is a relief' or 'At least we now know exactly what we are up against and what has to be done' (Brewin 1991). One recent study found 39% of patients recalled doctors communicating the diagnosis showed a less than caring attitude: they were perceived as uneasy, worried, rushed, arrogant or judgmental (Butow *et al.* 1996). The doctor needs to appear to have at least *some* idea of what it's like to be on the receiving end. Warmth, understanding and empathy are needed, and these probably come across better when they are transmitted nonverbally.

How Emotions Limit Communication and Understanding

Many patients are in shock when they first hear the word 'cancer', and very little may be remembered from the bad news consultation. Being in shock and failing to take in the information should not be confused with denial (Souhami 1978):

> *A 40-year-old woman had extensive Hodgkin's disease, which was fully explained to her and her husband by the medical registrar. 'I sat there and I could see him talking but I couldn't take anything in. When I got home I burst into tears, but afterwards I calmed down and my husband explained all that had been said'. A few weeks later, when I went over the treatment with her, she listened calmly and asked several direct, pertinent questions.*

Cassidy (1991) describes the process of breaking bad news as a modification of the history-taking method used by doctors more generally. By tracing the story of their illness step by step, the carer can get a reasonably clear idea of the patient's preferred coping strategy. This is important because it helps to dictate the pace and helps to gain the patient's confidence. There are a number of reasons why giving bad news tends to be difficult for health professionals: fear of being blamed, fear of the unknown and the untaught, fear of unleashing an emotional reaction, fear of expressing emotion, fear of not knowing all the answers and personal fear of illness and death (Buckman 1984; Espinosa *et al.* 1996). Some people choose careers in medicine in order to acquire the sense of invulnerability, of walking among the sick while remaining healthy. It is important to be aware of one's own fears about illness and death if one is in the position of breaking bad news.

Fear of causing pain and taking away hope, fear of facing therapeutic failure and conflicts around a decision to withhold the truth already taken by one's superiors are three more reasons why breaking bad news may be difficult for individual doctors (Buckman 1986). Another set of factors derives from the fact that if doctors do begin to talk about the bad news, they may feel pushed into assuming responsibility for the disease itself, and they may become more identifiable as the target for blame rather than as allies of the patient. Some doctors shield patients from the full truth, hoping that an optimistic picture will hearten the patient. It may also be tempting to take the credit when there is a remission and agree, even tacitly, that the patient has been cured. Also, exerting control over the information may not alter the clinical prospects for the patient but it may serve to protect the doctor (Buckman 1986). In response to bad news, a patient may burst into unconsolable crying, become panic-stricken in the clinic, shout at staff in an uncontrollable rage, or scream out distress. Other patients become silent and withdrawn or evidence disbelief. Still others take the news apparently calmly and matter-of-factly and experience their emotional reaction when they get home, sometimes much later. Unpleasant physical sensations or altered behaviours associated with acute anxiety and panic may also occur, and these may be distressing in themselves (Worden 1983). When these symptoms appear in the short term, they are features of normal grief and are not in themselves abnormal. They are nonetheless very painful feelings for staff to respond to and may cause staff as well as patients considerable distress (Maguire 1975):

> *The feeling is just indescribable. Unless you've experienced it you just don't know ... I was just so frightened. All I could think of was the children. If anything is going to happen to me, they are still so young.*

Beginning the process of disclosing bad news can be achieved by what Buckman (1989) calls *'the warning shot'*. For example, the doctor may have a suspicion on clinical examination that a growth may be more than benign and may sow the seeds of this idea by saying 'Well, it's probably a cyst, but we'll remove it and have a look', in other words conveying in a cautious way to the patient that there is a possibility that it could be more sinister and perhaps gently to introduce this idea to them as something to think about. The next step may occur at the point where biopsy results are known, 'Well, we've taken a look and it wasn't quite so simple as we first thought'. Giving a warning shot can involve the sort of remark that opens up to the patient the notion that 'all is not as straightforward as we'd hoped'. Buckman also uses a technique called 'aligning' where rather than telling the patient bluntly what is wrong, they are asked for their own opinion about the problem and what they think is happening. This may then allow the doctor gently to confirm the fact of the diagnosis.

According to Maguire and Faulkner (1988b,c) the key is to *slow the whole process down* so the transition for patients from being well to being seriously ill can be absorbed at their own pace. A number of general aims are worth bearing in mind:

- to get information across and to clarify that it has been understood

- to allow patients to consider their options and participate in the decision-making process

- to determine the emotional impact of what has been said

- to allow the patient enough time to ventilate worries

- to be aware of psychological defences and to be able to distinguish these from genuine misunderstanding

- to allow patients to limit what they want to know

- to know when to stop informing and when to listen

- to be empathic

- to be aware that patients will often be in a state of shock and not able to take in everything; it will be necessary to repeat things, ask about what has been understood and then repeat them again.

At the diagnostic stage, doctors need to be aware that they are the key figures from whom patients need support. As Holland and Jacobs (1986) point out, the doctor who is often the bearer of bad news must be prepared to accept in a supportive manner the patient's distress and sometimes hostility. It is also important not to break bad news and then switch immediately to advice-giving or reassurance. The patient needs time to respond emotionally to the news. It is important to be ready to hear strong emotions expressed. You are unlikely to hear patients' emotional concerns if you switch into advice-giving or reassurance.

Two case histories illustrate the dilemma of what to say to patients and families about bad news where the situation was complex and did not fit any easy set of guidelines. The first concerns **telling the prognosis**

> Mrs P, a woman in her thirties, was being treated for a brain tumour and was nearing the terminal phase of her illness. She was not moribund and although a new treatment was offered it was generally considered that only palliative treatment was realistic. Her family were adamant that her hopes about the experimental treatment be sustained so that she would not be upset by the reality of her poor prognosis. It was finally agreed that the subterfuge would be maintained. In due course the patient was transferred to a hospice where she became increasingly unclear in her thinking and any opportunity for open and honest discussion was lost. So too was the opportunity for this patient to put her emotional affairs in order and say her goodbyes.

The second history relates to **referral to the hospice**.

> Mr. D was being treated on the hospital ward for an advanced lung cancer and appeared to be totally failing to acknowledge the seriousness of his disease. This was considered by the nursing staff to be inappropriate because not only were they unable to raise with him any practical issues about his own wishes regarding further care but also it was creating substantial marital discord. The patient was complaining bitterly that they wanted to put him into a hospice to die and that his wife wanted to see him dead. An initial evaluation of this man's coping response suggested that he had been using denial or avoidance to deal with his fears. He talked a great deal at first about his symptoms. He eventually talked about the hospice, saying, 'That's where you go to die, isn't it?' He insisted they were consigning him to a 'wooden overcoat', when he himself felt he was far from dying. He began to talk about his fears, following which he was able to ask, 'Can you tell me what will happen when I go to the hospice?' to which it was

continued

continued

> possible to reply, 'They will help to make you comfortable and
> care for you in a way that may be more difficult to do here. They
> will try to understand your fears and be there for you'. – 'Can I go
> and visit to see what it is like?' he asked. Eventually he and his wife
> went to visit the hospice and together decided that he would go
> there.

For both of these patients there were issues about telling the
truth, about the amount of information they wanted, their
coping strategies and the impact of this on their behaviour and
levels of distress. Above all else they illustrate the need to
listen to what patients want to know and allow them to lead
the discussion of bad news. The way to do this is to follow the
patient's lead, refrain from offering advice too early, turn their
questions around so that rather than trying to find the answer
for them they are allowed to find their own solution, to watch
for clues in their behaviour that will tell you something about
what they are feeling and to give them plenty of time to come
out with what they really want to say and not rush in too
early to resolve the situation. Trying to find a way of solving
their problems is not the aim; rather, it is to provide a forum
in which they can work out their own solution, if possible. It
may be helpful when breaking bad news to follow the following basic principles.

- ensure there is somewhere to talk that is private without
  interruptions
- a degree of informality will help because it encourages
  people to ask questions and to feel free to express feelings
- check at each point that they have understood
- respond to questions truthfully and ask whether they
  want more information
- allow them to limit what they want to hear
- consistent eye contact helps to convey interest and a readiness to listen
- be aware of distancing tactics and avoid them

- ask open-ended questions (e.g. 'What do you think about this?') rather than closed questions (e.g. 'Do you think this is a good idea?'; closed questions require only a yes/no answer)

- don't be afraid to admit when you are out of your depth or have reached the limits of your skills

- it is often appropriate to have a close family member of the patient present at the time.

Patients are likely to be anxious and will not be able to take in quite a lot of what they are being told. An accompanying relative may take in different aspects of the information. Afterwards, they can pool the information they have or even clarify things with each other: 'I thought he said the treatment would make me feel ill'. – 'No, no, he said that it made some people feel sick for a short time afterwards but that it didn't usually last more than a couple of days'.

What patients say during the interview is usually an indicator not only of how much information they want but also of how they cope with hearing it. Therefore, it is crucial to listen to the message the patient is giving. For example:

> *Doctor*: 'I'm sure that it is very upsetting to hear that one moment you are healthy and the next you have a very serious illness. It would be understandable to feel upset. Do you want to talk about how you feel about your diagnosis?'
> *Patient*: 'No, I don't really want to talk. I just feel that I have to get over it. I'll be all right. I just need some time.'

This message is clear. However they may want to come back and talk at a later time and the door should be left open for this. The patient's behaviour also holds important clues to what they are thinking and feeling. Notice how you are feeling yourself and the impact the encounter is having on you. Try to resist the temptation to leave a difficult situation as soon as possible. Giving a piece of information that will completely change someone's life demands time, and this time should be given with good grace and perceived to be an integral part of one's professional responsibilities. In addition, technical terms and jargon may make you feel safe but it can mystify the patient.

The problem at the heart of breaking bad news concerns the needs of the *bearer* of that news, which is the desire both to protect the patient and be honest with them. Goldberg (1984) suggests that disclosure of bad news is a process and that it is often not possible to achieve this in a single or simple transmission. Denial and avoidance are powerful defences against something too awful to acknowledge. Through a series of questions, patients should gradually be led to reveal their experience of the illness and treatment process. The patient is allowed to maintain denial if necessary but is also invited to open up areas for more discussion. Others suggest that it is a physician's job to supply information in such a way that uncertainty can be optimally reduced and patients enabled to discuss their illness and treatment with people in their immediate environment in a sensible way (Molleman *et al.* 1984). Part of the skill in breaking bad news lies in clinicians' ability to make use of a 'window of opportunity' (Branch and Malik 1993), as illustrated below.

Wife of patient: He's having this treatment ... It's very new ... It's a new chemotherapy ... The doctor said he was very pleased with his progress.
Interviewer: What did the doctor say?
Wife: Well, I said if we could have a few years that would be all I want ... but he [the doctor] just patted me on the arm and looked at me...
Interviewer: He patted you on the arm?
Wife: I don't think it is a few years ... because he just looked at me. You know, it was just something about the way he [the doctor] looked at me.
Interviewer: He just looked at you?
Wife: I think he's only got a few weeks.
Interviewer: Are you saying that your husband's only got a few weeks?
Wife: Well, he hasn't got long ... I think the doctor was trying to tell me that he's dying ... In fact, if I'm honest I would say that I know he's dying.

Here the conversation has progressed from the wife seemingly saying she believed the chemotherapy would provide a long period of remission to admitting that her husband was indeed dying, without there having been any need to confront her about her initial unrealistic belief. Enabling is the process of picking up on the things that sneak through in the conversation, hinting that perhaps the bad news is known already or starting the process of gently introducing the notion that all is not well. In this example, the interviewer has made use of a reflective technique to facilitate the admission of knowledge of bad news. The original doctor used very powerful nonverbal methods – the touch and the look conveyed a message – and he had used his own window of opportunity at just the right time.

'Am I dying, Doctor?'

For many health professionals a real dilemma is presented by the terminally ill patient wanting to know their prognosis. Relatives may ask the same question about the patient. In some instances, the answer is clear in medical terms, 'Yes, they are certainly terminally ill', but the challenge is to say this to patients or relatives without appearing hard or insensitive. Many times doctors faced with this question see that every messsage, verbal and nonverbal, that comes with it is saying, 'Please, Doctor, let it be good news, don't tell me the bad news'. In many respects, the issues are similar to those encountered in breaking bad news, except that here we have the specific circumstance of the patient who is terminally ill to whom the answer in truth would be, 'Yes, and quite soon'. The first problem lies not with the patient but with those who are trying to help. The need to give something positive to the patient is immensely strong. The urge to want to say something positive needs to be recognized and throughly examined. We need to examine our motives and ensure that what we do is guided first and foremost by our judgment of what the patient wants rather than what we would prefer.

Don't hedge the issue ought to be a guideline, but having decided to be truthful, if that is what the patient wants, then the person will need support. In many instances this support will have to come from the doctor. By feeling confident about the ability to communicate, this process can become far less painful or time consuming than is sometimes assumed. Some patients do ask this question but do *not* want the truth. One way to make a judgment about whether this is the case is to learn how this person has dealt with crises in the past. The response of avoidance is such a powerful psychological defence that it tends to get used again each time something stressful occurs. If that has been their response in the past, it is likely to be so now. It can also be helpful to tackle this as a family issue, gathering the whole family and asking what they want to know. Facilitating family communication in a patient's last days can pose considerable challenges. As one relative so clearly expressed it, 'Death is a one shot exercise and if it is blown there is no second go at getting it right'.

Doctors need to examine their motives and seek to under-stand why they withhold information and what benefits there might be from doing this, either for patients or for themselves. 'I do not wish the patient to know this because the patient will be upset' might be interpreted as 'because it will also upset me'. To give bad news may mean admitting that the skills for maintaining health are inadequate. Dishonesty may be comforting to the physician because the illusion can be main-tained that more can be promised than is actually available. This is not to say that this response is commonplace – on the contrary – but knowledge of one's own motives and emotions and the part they play in the communication process is essen-tial to good communication skills.

Specific Communication Problems

Distancing techniques

Some professionals are concerned about becoming too emotionally involved with patients, and to avoid this they use distancing techniques. Such an attitude is more consistent with the biomedical model – the body as a machine, disease as machine breakdown and the doctor's task as machine repair –

than the biopsychosocial model of medicine (Engel 1977). One way distancing is achieved is by maintaining behaviour conveying professional status and by doing things allowing disengagement from unpleasant events and emotional involvement. Avoiding eye contact is by far the most obvious method, along with a formal posture and addressing people as 'Mr' or 'Mrs'. Patients may be encouraged to address doctors and nurses by formal titles and discouraged from exchanging pleasantries. Personal questions are discouraged although doctors may feel free to ask them for intimate details of their lives. The most extreme examples are doctors who sit on the opposite side of a desk from the patient, do not address the patient by name and rarely look at the patient. Doctors can also distance themselves emotionally from patients' problems by intellectualization: viewing the patient as a problem or case and examining that problem in a cold and rational way. Two illustrations are offered. First, the wife of a patient described her encounter with a hospital consultant.

Mrs F told the story of how her husband was asked to undergo a series of tests and they were seen by the consultant who talked about how and when the tests would be done. The wife was then telephoned about one week later and told that the results revealed cancer. When she asked about prognosis, the doctor told her that her husband probably had 6–12 months to live. The news devastated her but the doctor had been unable to see that by breaking it over the telephone, it had made it even worse for her to take this bad news. The use of the telephone to give bad news is the ultimate distancing technique.

The second illustration is taken from a poem by W. H. Auden (1976) and is eloquently expressed.

Mr. Rose he turned to his students,
Said, 'Gentlemen, if you please,
We seldom see a sarcoma
As far advanced as this.'

The tendency to focus on the physical illness and fail to respond to psychological distress is another distancing technique.

These techniques are picked up as a method of self-protection and they may be important in helping to maintain the ability to provide care for patients without becoming too upset by tragic events; however, they also dehumanize. We *can* look patients in the eye, we *can* call them by their name and we *can* convey warmth without it causing us great mental damage. We will serve patients better if we develop techniques that allow us to cope with the impact of their problems other than by the cold methods described above.

Closure

Showing people in a warm and empathic way that we have time to listen to their worries can cause difficulties when we wish to draw the meeting to a close. Up to this point we may have been doing things aimed at encouraging people to talk. But how many times after spending time with people, do they begin to tell the most important things when there are only five minutes left? Closure, therefore, presents some difficulties and requires some skill. First, it is possible to warn at the beginning of the encounter that it will be necessary to stop when time runs out. This makes it less awkward for both professional and patient when this occurs. Second, we can give the warning shot, 'We only have another five minutes left and so...' Another method to use is the summary:

> Can I just interrupt you there so I can see if I have understood the problem?
>
> It seems to me that there are a number of issues you have mentioned and perhaps I could just summarize what they are.
>
> Perhaps we could pause here and see where we've got to.
>
> It's helpful for me, at this point, to just go through what you have been saying in order to see if I have a clear picture.

This type of remark conveys a number of things. It lets the person know that you need to take stock of what has been said and you need a space in which to do this. It also says you have been listening and allows them time at the end of their session to say whether your interpretation of events is correct. Summarizing can be done at a number of points throughout an encounter but is particularly helpful as a method of closing the session. In some instances, the patient may ignore these cues and wish to continue talking. It is acceptable to actually say, 'I'm afraid we're running out of time although, perhaps because this is so important, we should come back and talk about it in more detail next time we meet', or 'We do need to wind up now but I wonder if we could come back to this next time and give ourselves some more time to talk about it'.

Guidelines for Information-giving

Essential information for patients includes at least five elements:

- what investigations are to be done and what will they involve?
- what did the investigations show?
- what is the diagnosis?
- what is the treatment to be?
- what is the outlook?

A checklist of information given can be attached to the front of patients' medical notes so that all staff in contact with the patient know what information has been shared with the patient and relatives (Fletcher 1973; Bunston *et al.* 1993). A question promptsheet encouraging patients to ask what they wish to know may improve patients' ability to ask about the prognosis of their cancer (Butow *et al.* 1994). Audiotape recordings of the bad news consultation have also been found to be helpful by many cancer patients and their families (Ford *et al.* 1995).

Especially when the news is bad, the feeling person inside the patient needs to be uppermost in helpers' minds. There are unfortunately still some doctors and nurses who, when they perform an investigation or procedure, whether it be sigmoidoscopy, blood sampling or biopsy, treat the patient as if to say, 'If you would be so kind as to vacate your body while I perform this procedure...' Procedures are performed on patients who need respect, empathy and care. Doctors can improve communication with patients if they ask the patient to write down the instructions they have been given, avoid jargon and check to see that explanations have been understood. It also helps to use pamphlets for specific problems and remember that friendliness as an intervention is insufficiently appreciated (Fletcher 1973). The following guidelines (Morrow *et al.* 1983) are also useful in getting messages across clearly:

- give specific, definite advice rather than abstract, obscure suggestions
- categorize the information: what is wrong, what tests will be done, what treatment will be needed, what you can do to help yourself and what will happen in the long term
- repeat the information
- present the most important information first
- stress the importance of the instructions or advice
- use short words and sentences.

Before leaving the issue of information given to cancer patients, one piece of information that is seldom addressed is the **cause** of the disease. 'The person is really asking: "Why me? What did I do that caused me to get sick?"' (Cassell 1976) When this question is not answered by the doctor, the answer will be filled in by the patient. Patients in a recent breast cancer study had a wide variety of explanations for their illness ranging from stress, breastfeeding, having babies, being childless, living with cats, taking the birth control pill or using a banned weedkiller for an infestation of horsetails (Burton and Parker 1995). The patient *may* fill in the blank the doctor leaves with an unhelpful explanation, especially one involving self-blame. The answer to what causes many cancers is usually 'We don't know', but this uncertainty is seldom acknowledged unless the patient presses the point.

Informed Consent

Informed consent to cancer surgery or treatment is not 'just another piece of paper to sign'. Staff who work on surgical wards often do not appreciate the extent to which patients are handing over their intact bodies to be mutilated by disfiguring surgery. Full descriptions of the operation or treatment and its side effects should be given. If the patient asks for explanation, this should be provided by a member of the surgical or medical team and, if necessary, by the consultant. Informed consent documents should be written to reflect the reading ability of the average person (Grossman *et al.* 1994). Short words and short, declarative sentences should be used. It should be possible for patients to critique the forms, and some patients may wish to take them home before signing them. An example of a simple informed consent document is given that is within the very easy range of comprehension (Morrow *et al.* 1983). For example, the format B could replace that in A.

A. Your signature below constitutes your acknowledgment (1) that you have read and agreed to the foregoing, (2) that the proposed operation(s) or procedure(s) have been satisfactorily explained to you and that you have all the information that you desire, and (3) that you hereby give your authorization and consent.

B.
- What is to be done has been clearly explained to me.
- I have all the information I want about the operation(s) or procedure(s).
- I want to have the operation or procedure done.

I signed below because I agree with the above three statements.

Discussing Therapeutic Options: Giving Patients Choice

Not all patients want to be involved in treatment decisions, but an increasing number of patients do. Schain (1990) describes four response styles in breast cancer patients.

Type I: 'You decide for me, Doctor'

- most often an older woman accustomed to seeing doctors as the authority
- will do best with a doctor who describes options but takes the major role in decision-making

Type II: 'I demand you do the X procedure'

- more often a younger and more medically sophisticated woman
- may have already obtained a good deal of relevant information and may arrive at the consultation with the decision already made
- may present problems for the doctor who has difficulty with patients being so assertive or demanding, or who feel the treatment requested is not appropriate

Type III: 'I can't decide, Doctor'

- patient feels overwhelmed by the diagnosis and the options available and feels unable to make a decision
- may profit from counselling from a psychologist, liaison psychiatrist, counsellor or nurse specialist
- doctor should aim to contain the anxiety so decision-making ability is improved

Type IV: 'Given the options, your recommendations and my preferences, I choose X'

- benefits from as much information as possible
- wants her wishes to be respected, but also has regard for the doctor's expertise
- will be responsible for carrying through with treatment because of the joint nature of the decision.

Doctors typically experience great difficulty when a patient obstinately refuses a life-saving procedure. Useful questions to ask when this becomes a problem include (Himmelhoch *et al.* 1970):

- Do I fully understand the patient's reasons for the refusal?

- Do I have all the necessary diagnostic information?

- Does the patient fully understand what is wrong and what is being proposed to correct it?

- Does the family know what is going on?

- Is there agreement among the staff as to the optimum treatment plan for this patient? (Some patients will use staff disagreement about treatment as a reason to refuse consent.)

- What is the social and philosophical context in which the patient has refused the procedure? (Refusals may be based on religious or cultural grounds.)

- Is there some need for a change of approach to the patient? (Some patients require more choice than others.)

- In this case, are the procedures offered really necessary or the only alternative?

7
Counselling over the Course of the Illness

The Onset of Cancer in Context

Patients coming into hospital may have many other concerns besides cancer: retirement, moving house, bereavement, a partner's new job, financial problems, work stress, serious illness in a relative or problems with children. Sometimes cancer is only the latest development in a disastrous string of stressful life events.

> *First I lost my husband, then my son was killed in a car accident, my mother is dying of leukaemia, my daughter's husband has just walked out on her, my best friend moved away three months ago, and now this.*

Life events that may cause additional stress include problems in intimate relationships, previous grief reactions, marital conflict, unresolved childhood issues, family problems, psychiatric illness, childrens' crises and illnesses other than cancer (Vachon 1985). It can be a very supportive intervention to discuss with patients the onset of the disease in context. The helper is then responding not only to problems involved in adjusting to cancer but to the *whole* person who has been experiencing a sequence of life events, only the most recent of which is cancer.

It is not uncommon for cancer patients to present with problems of unresolved grief when they are admitted to hospital at the time of diagnosis. Sometimes the unresolved issues go back to childhood. These may involve unmourned losses of parental figures or a lack of nurturing from parents during formative years (Vachon 1987):

> When children have not known the consistent presence of a caring and secure parent or when such a relationship has been lost, children may be at risk of experiencing feelings of inadequacy and insecurity as adults in all of their close relationships.... Early parental losses or strained interpersonal relationships in early childhood may leave adults susceptible to depressive episodes when confronted with later adult loss experiences. These losses may evoke a regressive return to the earlier loss experience and the re-emergence of earlier self-images and role relationship models.

In some studies, a combination of loss events and a response of 'giving up–given up' in the face of these stresses has been found to predate the onset of cancer (Engel 1968). Not every cancer patient has such a history, but it is useful to be aware of the possibility that this story may be a feature in individual patients. Unresolved grief may, in some cases, complicate an individual's ability to deal with the current crisis and may markedly affect the course of the cancer. Factors affecting the nature of the grief reaction include who the lost person was, the nature of the attachment, the mode of loss or death, losses experienced in childhood, the patient's personality type and social support. When grief concerns a parent who died of the same disease, the patient may have developed a deep identification with that parent and their mode of death. In these cases, it is important to understand as fully as possible the details, because the patient may be operating under the assumption that their fate will be the same. Unresolved grief reactions may take the following forms (Worden 1983).

- chronic and prolonged: grieving never comes to a satisfactory conclusion
- delayed: a relative absence of grief early, but a reaction at a later point
- exaggerated: a reaction that is excessive and disabling; a person who 'cannot live without the other'

- masked grief: physical or emotional symptoms instead of overt grief.

Some of these patients may need to be referred for psycho-therapy. Unusually intense grief reactions and anticipatory grief reactions may be seen in patients who were sexually abused as children, especially when the cancer affects genital or reproductive organs. Generally speaking, the more self-blame is involved, the more intense the reaction. Intense anger and mistrust toward health care staff are also frequently seen and represent anger displaced from abusers or from mothers who failed to protect their children from abuse (Clark *et al.* 1990).

In families of cancer patients, the loss or impending loss of a parent prompts a review of the parent–child relationship by surviving adult children. In general, the more conflict-ridden and ambivalent these relationships, the greater the difficulty in managing grief. As is the case with cancer patients who were abused as children, reactions of anger in some relatives may be very strong, and part of this anger may be unhelpfully displaced onto health care staff.

Cancer Recurrence

The existential crisis of having cancer is repeated whenever a patient who was previously in remission has a recurrence. Breast cancer patients have been most frequently studied. Early-stage disease can be controlled for many years with surgery and adjuvant therapy before reappearing, and it may go through several cyles of remission and recurrence. Some patients develop a hypochondriacal preoccupation during remission, fearing recurrence above all else and misidentifying benign bodily symptoms. When recurrence happens, it can be a more distressing experience than the initial diagnosis (e.g. Northouse *et al.* 1995). Symptoms of anxiety and depression may recur along with the cancer, especially if the patient is experiencing other stressful life events. If a patient's life situa-tion has deteriorated in the intervening years, recurrent cancer may be many times more stressful than at diagnosis. Conflict between patient and partner can sometimes be acute at this time, especially if the patient wants to forego treatment this time and the partner puts strong pressure on the patient to comply (Brewin and Sparshott 1996). Those who are prone to blame medical staff for the illness often do so now, especially if more aggressive treatment is recommended or the patient is in a lot of pain. Doctors may be rebuked with questions like, 'You knew this was going to happen, didn't you?' and the patient and family may believe medical staff were dishonest with them about the prognosis. The sword of Damocles has come down, and someone must be to blame. Some cancer patients who did not need counselling at diagnosis can derive great benefit from it at times of recurrence.

Spiritual Needs of Cancer Patients

At every stage of the illness, the spiritual needs of cancer patients may go unrecognized. When the cancer is diagnosed or at times of recurrence, Biblical themes of suffering may come to mind for some patients: suffering as the lot of human-kind, as a punishment, a test, an atonement or a liberation. The sufferer's response may be linked to other Biblical themes, as in the sufferer as accepting, or the sufferer as victim (Atkinson 1993). Spiritual distress can present as guilt or anger (Faulkner and Maguire 1996).

Spiritual issues occur throughout the illness. There are patients who say they have no reason to go on living, who question the meaning of suffering and death, express despair or despondency or describe a loss of faith in God; patients who describe ambivalent feelings toward God, resentment toward God, or fear of God's anger; patients who do not discuss their feelings about dying with significant others; who express guilt feelings or confess thoughts and feelings associated with shame. These patients are all confronting spiritual issues (Highfield and Cason 1983). The recognition that problems such as these are spiritual in nature is a first step in referral to a member of the clergy, if that is desired by the patient. It can be counter-productive to call on clergy *only* at the point of death. An unfamiliar person who has obviously been called because death is imminent can be frightening to patients. Far better to involve clergy at the earliest possible stage.

Religious faith can provide support, solace and personal meaning during a crisis, and some patients turn to their spiritual roots during life-threatening illness. God may be seen as a partner with the patient in problem-solving, as the responsible party on whom the patient waits or as the unseen force who gives them skills to solve their own problems. Some pray for a miracle or seek faith healing, while others read spiritual texts or focus on the next life. Some review what they have achieved spiritually in this life; others spend long periods in prayer; still others turn to clergy or members of their congregations. The crisis of cancer may be positively reframed by religious people in at least three ways: each person has a unique spiritual destiny, no one will be given more than they can handle, and misfortune and suffering provide special opportunities for spiritual growth. All of these coping styles may be adaptive for particular patients. Asking whether patients are religious is less useful than asking how they view the spiritual significance of cancer and how religion is part of their healing process (Jenkins and Pargament 1995).

It has been said that 'most patients die as they have lived: some, with metaphysical and religious concerns on their minds; others, with the everyday preoccupations they have always had' (Osler 1906, quoted in Peteet 1985). As death approaches, questions of ultimate concern usually make their appearance if they have not already done so. If there are doubts about an afterlife, an anxiety state can result. To dismiss these by saying, 'These patients are anxious and depressed but that's natural, they're dying', may deprive them of a vital opportunity to come to terms with spiritual or faith issues. Some patients who have lost a childhood faith during their adulthood regain it during a life-threatening illness. Others may experience a shattering loss of lifelong faith. The meaning of life in spiritual or philosophical terms may become the focal concern of some patients. However, evangelizing doctors, clergy and fellow-patients can be a problem. Nursing staff should be aware if patients are feeling uncomfortable but lack the confidence to handle the situation.

There may be a need to intervene to protect the patient from this insensitive behaviour.

The Dying Patient

Doctors, it is sometimes said, spend their careers preserving life, and their dread of death may lead them to avoid the dying patient. Some consultants look after the dying by telephone, via their junior staff or through contact with relatives and nurses. If the patient complains, the doctor orders something for pain but seldom appears at the bedside. Care of the terminally ill patient is improving, but dying in general hospitals often leaves a great deal to be desired. Among younger staff there is often a deep sense of dismay at the quality of psychological care in hospitals but they often know they have poor training to help, and they frequently feel powerless to do anything for the dying patient.

An important issue is respecting the stage at which the patient is functioning as death approaches. It is as if there is a 'funnel' over the dying patient's bed: the field of the patient's interest grows increasingly narrow until it is only dying that matters. For awhile early on, for example, the Wimbledon tennis tournament may interest the patient, then only events in the family, then only the disease and perhaps pain, and then only dying, which, in the last moments, is done alone. No one else can do the patient's dying for them. In this final stage there is an acute sense of separateness from others. Not to recognize this and to ask a dying patient to speak about Wimbledon when that subject has ceased to be important is insensitive and unhelpful, although it may help the helper who cannot cope with the patient's feelings. Some patients have an acute need for company at various stages during the dying process. Others have more need for solitude. People are different and this, too, should be respected.

The whole of existence is *now* to the dying person. This immediacy of the present moment was movingly expressed in the playwright Dennis Potter's last interview on UK Channel Four Television in 1994. Potter, dying of cancer of the pancreas, spoke of seeing the blossom outside his window in

Ross-on-Wye during the last weeks of his life, his final spring (Channel Four Television 1994).

> We're the one animal that knows we're going to die, and yet we carry on paying our mortgages, doing our jobs, moving about, behaving as though there's eternity in a sense, and we tend to forget that life can only be defined in the present tense, it is, is, is. And it is now, only. As much as we would like to call back yesterday and indeed ache to sometimes, we can't. It's in us, but it's not there in front of us ...
>
> The only thing you know for sure is the present tense. And that nowness becomes so vivid to me that in a perverse sort of way, I'm almost serene, I can celebrate life. Below my window in Ross, when I'm working in Ross now at this season, the blossom is out in full. There's a plum tree. It looks like apple blossom but it's white. And looking at it, instead of saying, 'Oh that's nice blossom', now, last week, looking at it through the window when I'm writing, it is the whitest, frothiest, blossomiest blossom that there ever could be, you know.
>
> And things are both more trivial than they ever were and more important than they ever were. And the difference between the trivial and the important doesn't seem to matter. But the nowness of everything is absolutely wondrous, and if people could see that, there's no way of telling you, you have to experience it, the glory of it, the comfort of it, the reassurance ... The fact is that if you see the present tense, boy, do you see it, and boy, can you celebrate it, you know?'

Feelings of this intensity often emerge among the dying, although they are perhaps seldom so eloquently expressed. Helpers can help the dying according to the extent of their own development, the degree to which they have faced their own mortality, and their ability to attend to and cope with their own and the patient's feelings. Helpers' needs to reassure themselves or talk about something more cheerful can do real damage to the patient who wants to talk about dying. Potter said he had not shed a tear since being given his diagnosis, but to have someone to cry with is cherished by some patients more than anything – and by some, the tears of others are more precious than their own. Visitors to the bedside of the dying often feel helpless, but there are great benefits in simply 'sitting with' patients. Silence goes far beyond words at such times. Health professionals are often profoundly uncomfortable with silence – they have to feel they are *doing* something, and this may be one of the most important lessons learned by those who wish to counsel the dying.

Cassidy (1986) describes the range of feelings found among dying patients:

> *Fear.* We are all afraid of illness, death and the unknown. Families and carers alike often try to protect someone they love from this fear by concealing the truth ... More common than the fear of death, however, is the fear of dying horribly.
>
> *Loss.* The whole of life is a series of losses, of letting go, of little deaths, and this is greatly accelerated in a terminal illness.
>
> *Anger.* Anger against fate or against God needs to be voiced and accepted, not met with pious explanations or platitudes ... Less easy to cope with is anger against medical colleagues. It is an unpalatable fact that some patients are misdiagnosed or badly handled ... Mistakes admitted are usually forgiven ... The bitterest anger against doctors ... is not because of failure of diagnosis but of lying. I remember well the anguished sobs of a young man with an oat cell tumour of the lung as he cried out loud, not 'I am going to die', but 'He lied to me. He lied to me.' This betrayal was more painful than the prospect of death.
>
> *Alienation.* Surrounded by false reassurances, the patient feels guilty about saying how ill he feels or expressing his fears and gradually withdraws ... The condition of loneliness is further compounded by alienation of the patient from his medical carers. In the face of cheerful reassurance and evasive answers, he is humiliated into silence.

An excellent resource for those who care for the dying is Charles-Edwards' *The Nursing Care of the Dying Patient: In the Midst of Life* (1983). Patients who have witnessed a death on the ward may wish to speak about it, and staff need to be prepared to speak openly with them. Charles-Edwards vividly describes the defences that come into play among some health care staff who treat the dying:

> *Most members of the caring professions, particularly nurses and doctors, find it all too easy to hide behind the cloak of busyness ... The district nurse who bustles in, rushes through a blanket bath and dressing at a rate of knots, chattering cheerily away throughout, is saying quite clearly that she has no time to listen. The family doctor who never visits his terminally ill patients unless specially requested to do so, and when he does, keeps his coat on, rarely lifts his eyes from his prescription pad and leaves the house in five minutes flat, is giving the same message. It happens with even greater frequency in hospital, when the consultant, complete with his entourage of students, housemen and registrars performs his ward round ... When the ward round reaches the dying patient, many consultants will merely acknowledge his presence by a courtesy greeting as they pass the foot of the bed. The rest of the team, following his lead, will either talk amongst them-*

selves as they walk by, or else throw the patient an embarrassed, apologetic smile.

The dying patient may thus come to feel increasingly isolated, and opportunities for helping are missed.

Communication with Dying Patients

We discussed in Chapter 6 the dilemmas posed to health professionals by the questions, 'How long will I live?' and 'Am I dying, Doctor?' A third and equally difficult question is 'What will it be like?' by which the patient may be asking, 'What can I expect to experience in my final days of life?' As Creagan (1994) observes, behind this question may lie a specific concern. It is helpful to ask what exactly is meant by this question: 'What concerns you? What is the overriding problem that troubles you at the moment?' Some patients may be fearful of dying in the way a loved relative died. Others may be worried about choking, haemorrhaging, hallucinating or behaving irrationally in their final hours. Helpers may need to ask specifically about individual patients' concerns.

An issue that often arises as the terminal stage approaches is whether patients should be told they are dying. What is difficult here is that patients have both a right to know and a right not to know, if they choose to remain ignorant of their condition. Kubler-Ross (1969) described five stages in death and dying – denial, anger, bargaining, depression and acceptance – but these are not stages to 'push' a patient through. Some patients never get beyond denial. Information should be given to patients as and when they are ready to receive it. Patients should dictate both the pace and the degree of openness.

Physical contact may be very helpful, but if the helper's manner says 'I am afraid of you' or 'Do cheer up and talk about jolly things', the patient's trust is not going to be won. When a difficult question is asked, one that may have a painful answer, averted eyes or a look of embarrassment or anxiety will make the patient suspect a dishonest answer. The dying patient is exquisitely sensitive to nonverbal communication. It is important to remember that even when unconscious the patient may continue to be aware of sound and touch, and there is sometimes an awareness of the presence of other people in the room. It may be important to explain to the unconscious patient and hold their hand in the same way as you would with a conscious patient and encourage relatives to do the same. Charles-Edwards (1983) provides this excellent example of the supportive provision of information to a dying patient.

Arthur: It's lung cancer, isn't it?

Sister: How long have you known?

Arthur: Ever since I first went to the doctor, when my voice started getting husky and the coughing started. How long have I got, Sister?

Sister: Thank goodness, that's one question no one can answer for you.

Arthur: Can't you give me any idea?

Sister: Well, I would say weeks rather than days or years, but there's really no telling for sure.

Arthur: (weeping now for the first time) God, I'm scared. It's not dying that's so bad, but how it will happen. The pain's been so bad sometimes that I've longed to be dead time and time again over the last twelve months.

Sister: Arthur, I've never lied to you before and I'm not lying now. I promise that when the time comes it won't be nearly as bad as you're imagining. You'll just get very weak and gradually sleepy, not suddenly, but over a few days. The pain will almost certainly get less severe, it nearly always does, but if you have any pain, we can give you drugs to stop it. I promise that you won't die in pain and I promise that someone will be with you all the time.

Arthur: (wept for five or ten minutes letting the Sister comfort him) I shall have to tell my wife what you've told me, that it's cancer and everything.

Sister: As I think you'd guessed, your wife does know.

Arthur: I'll give her hell for keeping it from me.

Sister: Why do you think she's kept it from you?

Arthur: ''Cos it's too painful to talk about. (tears again) ... Well, thank you for being so straight with me. That's what I really like about you.

In broaching the topic of fatal illness with patients, it may be helpful to say, 'Perhaps you have been wondering how seriously ill you are', and if the patient answers no, 'Well, perhaps we should look at this' or 'Tell me how you understand what has been upsetting you' (Cramond 1970).

Dubovsky and Weissberg (1982) suggest the following general guidelines for communicating with dying patients.

- Be truthful with the patient and answer questions directly.

- If patients do not seem to understand the diagnosis, they may not be ready to accept the news that it is a fatal illness. When they are ready, they will begin to ask questions.

- Some patients continue to deny awareness of the seriousness of their illness until the day they die. Usually, little is gained by confronting this denial.

- Treat pain with adequate doses of narcotics.

- Accept the range of emotional reactions experienced by patients and discuss them openly.

- Do not discourage hope about the future even if it seems unrealistic.

- Avoid attempting to bolster false hope with empty encouragements such as, 'A cure for your disease might be just around the corner'.

- If patients are hospitalized, ask if they would like a roommate and, if so, provide one.

- Treat depression vigorously, as in a patient with a normal lifespan.

- Communicate the attitude that even though the dying patient cannot be cured, a great deal can be accomplished in what remains of life to add meaning and richness to it.

- Remember that most people die as they live and that dying brings out the best in some individuals and the worst in others.

Fletcher (1973) speculates about why health professionals are so reluctant to talk to the dying. He describes the resentment some doctors experience in turning aside to help their 'failures', passing by the end of the bed with an embarrassed nod, or giving a brief word of unconvincing encouragement. Talking to the dying is costly in time and emotionally demanding, and doctors have until recently had little or no training for the complex issues raised, emotional and spiritual.

They also tend to look on death as something that happens to patients and not to themselves. An essential part of a doctor's or nurse's training is coming to terms with their own mortality. Staff should offer time when the *patient* wants to talk. Not all patients wish to do so, and reticence needs to be respected. In hospital everyone tends to leave this task to someone else. The house officer and ward sister may be in the best positions to help, and the hospital chaplain can play a vital role. When patients are very depressed, a liaison psychiatrist may be helpful (Fletcher 1973).

The helper's emotional response to the dying is often sympathetic identification with their plight combined with feelings of inadequacy, lowered self-esteem and frustration. Denial, reluctance to discuss the illness with the patient and avoidance of the patient and his or her family may then follow (Gorlin and Zucker 1983). A number of strategies are suggested that may help health care staff cope with their negative emotional responses to the dying (Table 7.1).

The Dying Patient's Family

Perhaps more than at any other stage of the illness, care of dying patients intimately involves their family. Sometimes it is immediately clear that the strong feelings being expressed by a surviving partner are to do with an agreement between the couple that one of them was going to die first, except it isn't happening that way, and there are feelings of anger, betrayal and guilt. The existence of such agreements, spoken or unspoken, often move into the foreground as death approaches. Family conflicts of very long standing can make a reappearance, emotions may run high, and hospital staff may get caught in the crossfire.

Many relatives have conflicting feelings as death approaches. Some prefer to retreat behind a wall of denial and are unable to face the death squarely. Not infrequently, the patient expends energy in attempting to protect family members from the truth. Sensitive counselling can help to prevent this situation persisting over long periods. Family members can also create problems when they ask that the dying patient be protected from the truth. 'Often the family tells the doctor that

Table 7.1 Strategies to help health care staff cope with their negative emotional responses to dying patients

Helpers' emotional or behavioural reaction to dying patients	Suggested coping strategies
Avoidance	Attempt to understand the feelings that lead to avoidance; stay with the patient; discuss with colleagues
Identification with the patient	Recognize; avoid tendency to deny seriousness of disease or to give way to despair
Hostility/rejection	Acknowledge and analyse; if situation is intolerable, transfer patient to another physician
Feelings of inadequacy	Discover areas in which help and comfort can be given; be realistic about limitations of medicine
Feelings of loss of control or threatened authority	Acknowledge and analyse; be realistic about personal limitations and actual range of influence and authority
Frustration, confusion, uncertainty about dealing with the patient; coping strategies ineffective for the situation	Request consultation with clinical psychologist or liaison psychiatrist; consider referral of the patient
Anxiety, guilt and frustration about meeting patient's recognized emotional needs	Allocate time realistically according to need; request consultation or referral

the patient must not be told bad news because they "couldn't take it". In those situations the doctor is not sure who cannot take what, and it becomes necessary to make delicate inquiries as to where the problem lies' (Cassell 1976).

It is helpful when the family of the dying are seen not as adversaries but rather as part of the health care team. While the doctor or nurse is admitting the patient, another member of staff can take the next-of-kin into a private room and spend some time getting to know them. Family members often feel guilty at the time of hospital admission, feeling they have failed the patient in some way. Staff may observe anticipatory grief and much anxiety about the future. When relationships have been strained the problems are compounded, especially when there is guilt about feeling relief at the patient's imminent death. Whenever possible, family and close friends should be seen together and given information at the same time: problems can arise when there is disharmony or competition for information among those around the bedside. Communication between patient and family is crucial at this time, and anything staff can do to facilitate this will remove one burden from the patient.

One common problem is dealing with the conspiracy of silence between partners when one of them is dying. If possible, the counsellor should see them together. You might begin by saying you are aware how worried both of them have been about her illness (for example), but how it has been very difficult to broach the subject. You can understand why that is, because neither can bear to see the other hurt and upset. However you are also aware there are a lot of things they want to say to each other. He wants to be able to share her fears, and she wants to help him to begin to grieve and to make some preparation for the future. What seems to have stopped them both from talking openly has been that knowing she is dying and may not live for very much longer has been too frightening to share (Charles-Edwards 1983). It can be important that the words 'death' or 'dying' are used by the helper, so that neither the patient nor the relative is left to use the painful word for the first time.

There are several signs that patient and family have begun the **anticipatory grief** process. There is heightened anxiety, and intense emotions make their appearance. Profound sadness, guilt, anger and grief, accompanied by crying, are close to the surface and easily precipitated. There is increased attention to existential questions such as 'Why has this happened to us?' An acceleration of the life review process is seen in patient and family – the meaning of their lives and the significance of their relationships to one another. Alterations in the intensity of the patient–family bond begin to occur.

Patient and family may begin to disconnect from one another emotionally. Patients withdraw themselves from the lives of their families, and family members may unconsciously begin speaking of the patient in the past tense. Other families may rather desperately cling to the patient, which may be an indication of a troubled relationship or unresolved guilt. The patient's sense of time becomes compressed: 'by next Christmas' becomes 'if I make it 'til Christmas'. These are signals that the family and the patient have taken on board the medical reality and begun the process of mourning (Weisman 1979b, quoted in Hermann 1985).

Those counselling the patient should be ready to meet acute emotional distress in the patient's loved ones. Among these feelings are (Cassidy 1986):

- fear: of death, of pain and of dying badly; of not being able to cope, of letting their loved one down

- loss: a loved person fading before one's eyes, and the appearance of a sick person whose demands may be more than they can cope with

- anger: against God, fate, doctors and hospitals may be greater than in the patient, and may occur against disturbing treatments that fail to cure

- revulsion: however much a person is loved, a gross disfigurement, stinking wounds, vomit, sputum or excreta may make people feel revolted

- weariness: carers run out of energy and may find, to their dismay, that they are bored by caring for a sick person and want to get on with their lives; these feelings are rarely expressed because people assume they are unacceptable, and the problem is compounded by guilt; there is a need for respite from caring

- guilt: 'If only I'd made him go to the doctor sooner...'; there may be guilt about marital discord or infidelity, or about no longer being able to care for a loved one at home

- exhaustion: this work is demanding enough for professional nurses, but how much more demanding to care for an adored relative.

Psychological Adaptation to Death

Shock, denial, bargaining, anger, depression, fear, regression and resignation are all seen in the dying. They do not always occur in this order, and no patient should be 'pushed through the stages'. A fine and readable example of the story of one man's dying can be found in Morrison (1993). **Shock** is a kind of protective blanket that is thrown over us whenever emotions are aroused so violently that we might be overwhelmed by them. However sensitively patients are given information about terminal illness, they are almost certain to experience waves of shock. **Denial** occurs; as we observed in Chapter 3, it is almost never appropriate to attempt to force a person who is denying the truth to acknowledge it.

At the stage of **bargaining**, the patient asks for just a little more time – to see the birth of a grandchild, perhaps, or to attend a child's wedding. **Anger** is expressed at loved ones, at God and at medical staff. 'Why me, Where did I go wrong?' The counsellor needs to learn to listen to and feel the anger without defending against it with words. As anger subsides and denial and bargaining break down, **depression** creeps in: the pain of anticipated loss, sadness over those things never to be achieved, guilt and regret about pain caused to others during one's life, and the loss of safety as one approaches an unfamiliar void. Insomnia, anorexia and weakness may leave the patient weary of life. Tears flow most readily now. The helper needs to permit and encourage the sharing of distressing thoughts and feelings – it is never possible or appropriate to try to 'cheer up' a depressed person. Sadly, many patients remain in this state of depression until they die.

Fear of the mode of dying and of the life (or lack of it) to come is almost universal and is often worse at night. Men are often reluctant to admit that they are afraid because they see this as unmanly or a sign of weakness. Many believers are ashamed to acknowledge their fears about death and dying, and it may fall to a member of the clergy to give permission and encouragement to express these feelings. **Regression** to a childlike dependency can be a defence against working through grief. Patients who have lived through traumatic experiences in the past may experience nightmares or flashbacks. Some patients respond to loss of control by becoming obsessional, preoccupied with the arrangement of possessions and papers around the bed – constantly rearranging them, moving things back and forth half an inch. Some patients throw a temper tantrum if their favourite nurse does not bath them on a given day.

Resignation is far more likely than full acceptance of impending death. Some patients never reach a stage of peace and can be angry, denying and fighting until they die. Some grow increasingly distressed, making life almost unbearable for their families and those caring for them. Some welcome death, and this group includes those severely weakened by illness, the elderly who have grown weary of life, those with exceptional faith and those whose lives have been so miserable that death represents an end to suffering. On the one hand, the transition into unconsciousness may be almost imperceptible for some. On the other hand, some go through anguish in their final hours that is very difficult for their loved ones to bear (Charles-Edwards 1983). Quill (1995) movingly describes the bad death as a medical emergency. One patient whose pain could not be adequately controlled in his final days rebuked his physician with the words, 'You promised me I wouldn't die like this!'

'To watch another human being die can be an extremely intense learning experience. Those who have the opportunity to serve a dying person physically, psychologically or spiritually may experience some of the most profound of human emotions' (Garfield 1976). However the emotional demands on the team caring for the dying patient require attention. This is stressful work. It is emotionally draining. Staff need good health, good relationships outside work, and emotional and spiritual support. When this work is done well it has costs to helpers. Mount (1986) offers useful advice on how to recognize occupational stress and deal with it in the team.

Bereavement

Relatives may experience a spectrum of feelings in bereavement. There may be muted feelings, great sadness or overwhelming desolation; however, the pleasure and relief that are expressed in some cases may be more difficult for staff to manage. For a financially dependent partner there may be loss of a lifestyle, and for a disabled partner bereavement may mean a move into an institution. The stages of working through grief resemble those of the dying patient already discussed: shock, acute grief, denial and searching, imaginary conversations with the deceased, illusions of the dead person's presence, vivid dreams of the deceased, guilt, anger, depression, loneliness and, finally, resolution. Worden's (1983) book on grief counselling is an excellent text for anyone who wishes to help relatives of cancer patients in their bereavement. He describes four tasks of mourning:

- to accept the reality of the loss (versus denial of the loss)
- to experience the pain of grief (versus not to experience this pain)
- to adjust to an environment in which the deceased is missing (versus not adapting)
- to withdraw emotional energy and reinvest it in another relationship (versus holding onto the past attachment and not forming new ones).

Mourning is finished when the four tasks of mourning are accomplished. Usually one to two years are required, although no definite limits can be set. Working through grief may be a long-term process. Grief counselling is to facilitate the processes of normal grief, whereas grief therapy is about resolving pathological grief. The following are clues to disturbed grief reactions and suggest the need for a psychotherapy referral (Worden 1983).

- chronic grief reactions (prolonged and unresolved)
- delayed grief reactions (a postponement of grieving)

- exaggerated grief reactions (an intensification of grief)
- masked grief reactions (physical symptoms that are the equivalent of grief)
- the person cannot speak of the deceased without experiencing intense and fresh grief
- an intense grief reaction triggered off by some relatively minor event
- themes of past losses come up in an interview about the deceased
- there is an unwillingness to move material possessions belonging to the deceased
- friends or activities associated with the deceased are excluded
- a long history of subclinical depression with persistent guilt and low self-esteem
- a compulsion to imitate the dead person
- self-destructive impulses
- unaccountable sadness occurring at a certain time each year
- a phobia about illness or death.

The bereaved have an increase in mortality from all causes, and some relatives will be more at risk than others for disturbed grief reactions. Those who were insecurely attached to their parents in childhood, who were ambivalently or dependently attached to the deceased, who have low self-esteem, low trust in others, a previous psychiatric disorder, previous suicidal gestures or attempts, and an absent or unhelpful family are at risk for complicated bereavement reactions (Parkes 1996). Some of these individuals can be identified and counselled early before problems become severe.

8
The Psychodynamic Model

This chapter describes two psychodynamic techniques that have been used with cancer patients, the psychodynamic life narrative and brief, focused psychodynamic therapy.

The Psychodynamic Life Narrative

In listening to the patient's story, it is often possible to begin to place the illness in the context of the patient's life history and current situation (Streltzer and Leigh 1978; Viederman and Perry 1980). For example:

> Shortly after you married you lost your mother, a newborn baby and your husband one after another. A road traffic accident also occurred about that time. The first marriage had been a good one, but when your husband died, you remarried hastily out of loneliness. Your second husband was violent and abusive. After 10 years of continued violence, even after the divorce, he was finally sent to prison, but then you lost the use of your legs as a result of the road traffic accident years before, until an operation helped you to walk again. You were no sooner beginning to resume a normal life than you developed breast cancer. Given all of these losses in your life, it is not surprising that you are feeling very depressed about the disease and about the operation. The cancer feels like a 'last straw'.

This is an extreme example of a life full of trauma, but patients often respond to such a formulation with the words, 'I never thought about it that way before, but it makes sense, doesn't it?' No attempt is made by the helper to alter the patient's coping style, but the current illness is placed in the context of the patient's overall life story and situation: 'Why me?' 'Why now?' 'Why this?' (Kleinman *et al.* 1978). Psychological problems, where present, become more understandable in the light of events. This relatively simple intervention can be of considerable comfort and support to the patient. The psychodynamic life narrative is a statement that places the physical illness in the context of the person's 'life trajectory'. It also offers a clarity and a logic to their emotional responses at a time when they may be struggling with hopelessness and a loss of control, and it communicates understanding. From a relatively brief intervention, there is the potential therapeutic impact of feeling understood.

The counsellor needs a sufficiently detailed psychosocial history to make sense of the patient's current plight. Areas to cover include:

- stories about the patient's conception (wanted/unwanted) and birth

- mother's miscarriages, stillbirths, babies that died, abortions and the patient's own terminations

- illnesses, accidents or separations as a child (include parents' illnesses/deaths, war trauma and serious illness or hospitalization in childhood)

- siblings: how many, what ages; how do you get on?

- mother's personality – how the patient got on with her as a child, her most difficult feature

- father's personality – how the patient got on with him as a child, his most difficult feature

- any 'nervous trouble' in parents, parents' families, siblings or self?

- school years: friends? academic performance? Follow up any traumatic events

- puberty: early/late? feelings about? Attitudes toward sexuality in the family (important where sexual problems are a feature)

- adolescence: first interest in opposite sex, first sexual experiences

- school leaving age: qualifications, academic career, career choice

- engagement, marriage or partnership, children, sexual adjustment, reproductive history

- relationships with partner, children, work colleagues

- adult bereavements: parents, siblings, friends, spouse (and ill health in significant others)

- menopause, empty nest syndrome, mid-life crises, retirement, other crises of adult life

- general prediagnosis health of patient, partner, surviving parents and children

- current life situation, hopes and aspirations, e.g. newly retired, recently widowed

- 'What was the most difficult time in your life? What got you through that?'

Two hour-long interviews or one hour-and-a-half interview may be required to gather the information needed for a psychodynamic life narrative. This psychosocial history is also needed for brief psychodynamic psychotherapy, which is discussed below. If questions about the patient's conception and birth appear curious, their importance lies in the early formation of a depressive life script, for example 'I wasn't wanted', 'I was a mistake' or 'My mother tried to do away with both her babies, and then I had an abortion in my teens. I think the cancer is punishment for what I did'. A diagnosis of cancer may be taken as a validation of self-concepts such as these: 'A fast-growing untreatable cancer is only what can be expected for someone like me'.

A key feature of the psychodynamic life narrative is the patient's history of previous loss events. In his popular book,

The Road Less Travelled, Scott Peck (1978) gives a useful list of what has to be given up at different stages of life in a normal life trajectory. The cancer patient facing a suddenly truncated lifespan may experience many of these losses at once, as if the tasks of several stages of life must be faced simultaneously and much more rapidly than is usual or feels bearable:

- the state of infancy, in which no external demands need be responded to
- the fantasy of omnipotence
- the desire for total (including sexual) possession of one's parent(s)
- the dependency of childhood
- distorted images of one's parents
- the omnipotentiality of adolescence
- the 'freedom' of uncommitment
- the agility, sexual attractiveness and/or potency of youth
- the fantasy of immortality
- authority over one's children
- various forms of temporal power
- the independence of physical health
- ultimately, the self and life itself.

The news that a person has or may have cancer affects the trajectory of future years, which once stretched indefinitely into the future. The emotions experienced at this time can be extreme and very distressing, especially for people who have had little previous experience of loss. There may be a number of losses involved:

- the loss of the notion that one enjoys perfect health: 'My body has let me down'
- the loss of an indefinite future stretching out ahead of one: 'How long do I have?'

- the loss of a sense of invulnerability and omnipotence: 'My lifespan is now limited'

- the loss of living to see one's children or grandchildren settled: 'I might not be here'

- the loss of hard-earned retirement years: 'Why now, of all times?'

- in the case of mutilating surgery, the loss of a body part or body function affecting body image and self-esteem: 'How am I going to feel without a breast?'

- the loss of security in a relationship: fears of losing one's partner's affection or sexual attentions because of mutilating surgery

- the loss of confidence in one's health: fears of ill health from the side effects of treatment.

There may also be unique and idiosyncratic losses an individual patient faces. For example: 'When I lost my first breast, my marriage was going through a bad patch. Now we have a wonderful sexual relationship, and I am going to have to lose the other breast. I feel absolutely devastated this time'. Some patients have an ill or handicapped family member to look after, and their first worry is for others. Other special circumstances in the life of the patient may create specific fears and concerns for an individual. These cannot be known until the patient's life situation is explored in detail. This can be a time-consuming task for the counsellor, but with practice counsellors can learn to listen for salient features in the history and develop the capacity to formulate key psychodynamic issues efficiently.

Brief Focused Psychodynamic Psychotherapy

Psychodynamic therapists make links between early childhood experiences and the patient's current character structure and symptoms. The patient's emotional response to the therapist (transference) and the therapist's emotional response to the patient (countertransference) are also sources of learning. Key patterns of feeling and behaving from early childhood are repeated or 'transferred' onto people in the patient's adult life, including the therapist. In **Malan's model** (1976), the triangle of insight (parent, therapist and current significant other) is interpreted to the patient each time it emerges in the material. For example, 'Given the pattern of rejection in your family, you came to expect that this was how you would be treated, so it was not surprising that you chose as a partner a man who would reject and demean you. Most recently you have come to expect that I will reject you by not offering you counselling'. There are as many variants of this interpretation of the triangle as there are focal interpersonal issues brought by patients.

Self-defeating patterns from childhood are often unconsciously re-enacted in adult life, and these patterns may have become focused around the cancer, for example, 'Nothing good happens to people like me', 'I must remain in control at all times' or 'Other people are not to be trusted'. Once this repetitive self-defeating pattern has been made conscious, there is the potential to achieve greater control over feelings and behaviour and avoid some of the repetitious negative outcomes of the past. Defence mechanisms are often a focus of interpretation in the psychodynamic model. A healthy respect on the part of the therapist for patients' needs to defend against painful or unwelcome material is important.

Another feature of psychodynamic therapy is the establishment of a secure holding environment (Winnicott 1965), one aspect of which is the provision of reliable boundaries. Sessions are conducted each week in the same place at the same time, and the therapist's punctuality, reliability, abstinence and confidentiality are integral parts of the therapeutic space. A major development in psychodynamic theory has been a shift away from Freud's emphasis on drives, drive derivatives and defence mechanisms toward an interpersonal or object relations base. (Paradoxically, objects in this context mean people. The original use of the term was that people in the patient's external world could become objects of the drives, eros and aggression.)

Psychodynamic psychotherapy may be conducted over

short- or long-term periods. Brief psychodynamic therapies have proliferated in recent years. The following inclusion criteria are fairly typical.

1. The patient must be suitable for long-term psychodynamic psychotherapy:
   - can respond to an interpretive approach
   - is able to work in the transference
   - has sufficient ego strength – no risk of ego diffusion or disintegration
   - no history of gross acting out, such as repeated suicide attempts or life-endangering behaviour
   - not currently heavily dependent on drugs or alcohol
   - no active psychosis or past psychotic episodes
   - no severe borderline personality disorders without psychiatric backup.
2. A psychodynamic focus can be found.
3. Circumscribed pathology exists.
4. The patient must be actively involved in object relations: no social isolates.

These criteria will tend to exclude patients with psychotic, chemically dependent, schizoid, psychopathic, narcissistic or borderline psychopathology. Also screened out will be those patients who, when asked to describe the problem, are unable to find a focus and reply, 'It's everything' (the problem of comorbidity). Such a patient may present with a collection of difficulties – marital and sexual problems, an eating disorder, chronic interpersonal conflicts, child-management problems, a history of depression and suicide attempts or the recent disclosure of sexual abuse in the family – and a recent diagnosis of [breast] cancer. The referring doctor may hear only about the last two events and conclude, 'Might be a suitable case for short-term counselling: looks like an adjustment reaction to recent trauma'; however, the rest of the history and diagnosis are missing and a detailed assessment needs to be done. Such patients should not be offered brief therapy and need longer-term work. Although described as 'brief', Malan's model consists of 20 sessions in the hands of an experienced therapist and 30 sessions when the therapist is inexperienced.

There are a number of brief psychodynamic psychotherapies in use at the moment, and this survey is necessarily selective. Crits-Christoph and Barber (1991), Groves (1996) and Messer and Warren (1995) give helpful overviews. One of the most popular models is Luborsky's **brief supportive-expressive psychotherapy** (Luborsky 1984) with its emphasis on the core conflictual relationship theme (CCRT), developed from an inspection of relationship episodes: the stories people tell about their interactions with other people. The CCRT is expressed as a sentence with two components: (a) a statement of the patient's wish, need or intention; and (b) a statement of the consequences of trying to get one's wish from another person. The CCRT is enacted in the triad of relationship spheres: (a) the therapeutic relationship; (b) current relationships outside therapy (family, co-workers, etc.); and (c) past relationships, especially with parents. These three domains of object relations are familiar from Malan's triangle of insight.

The focus of brief therapy is on a facet of the CCRT and the symptoms related to it. Luborsky represents the CCRT diagrammatically with three overlapping circles. In the centre, where the three circles overlap, is the CCRT. For example, the patient's wish is to receive love and affection but the repeated result of attempts to secure these is rejection. This pattern first appeared with parents (who could not respond emotionally to their child), then with a spouse or partner (who could not tolerate the patient's clinging dependency) and now with the therapist (who cannot grant the patient the out-of-hours contact that has been repeatedly requested). As in Malan's model, the basic pattern of the CCRT is made conscious and worked through in all three domains: parent, significant other and transference.

Strupp and Binder's (1984) **time-limited dynamic psycho-therapy** (TLDP) is an interpersonally focused treatment of 25–30 sessions or less. Early patterns of interpersonal relatedness, which originally served a self-protective function, are now seen to be anachronistic and self-defeating. These patterns recur in the therapeutic relationship, which serves as a laboratory for studying *in vivo* the patient's difficulties in living. The essence of the model is that patients suffer from the ill effects of previous interpersonal relationships and the therapist can provide a new experience, seeking to effect changes in the faulty learning the patient has carried forward from the past. A central issue or dynamic focus must be identifiable, and the patient must be able to form a collaborative relationship with the therapist because transference analysis is a major area of the work.

In this model, **internal object relationships** come into focus – self-images, images of the other and a set of transactions taking place between them. Enduring internal object relationships associated with strong emotions press for enactment in current interpersonal relationships including the therapeutic relationship, where they can be observed and discussed. The patient unconsciously seeks to draw from the therapist behaviours that re-enact the role assigned to the other in the patient's enduring scenario. The interpersonal relationship between therapist and patient oscillates between the valid adult–adult relationship of the present and the anachronistic child–parent relationship of the past.

The **dynamic focus** in TLDP is the central interpersonal story of the patient's life. In TLDP, the patient and therapist are engaged in a joint narration and renarration of the patient's central interpersonal dilemmas. Through this activity patient and therapist collaboratively author a new story with more flexible outcomes. The recognition of alternative stories and outcomes signals the beginning of therapeutic change. Practitioners of transactional analysis will find in TLDP echoes of Eric Berne's *life script* (1972).

A **12-session contract model** was devised by Mann (1973), who observed that all short forms of psychotherapy revive the horror of time, and therapists as well as patients have a will to deny this horror of time. The recurring life crisis of separation–individuation is the theoretical base upon which this therapy rests. All human beings are susceptible to re-experiencing the anxiety of the separation–individuation crisis at times of loss, and mastery of separation anxiety becomes a focus in this model. The patient is offered a statement about the nature of the central difficulty, which is both a formulation of the problem and a goal for treatment. The *central issue* is couched in terms of feelings and/or maladaptive function, is derived from childhood experience and continues into the present. Another ingredient of the central issue addresses the patient's **present and chronically endured pain** and often begins with the phrase, 'All your life, you...'. Usually this statement does not meet with denial; indeed it often provokes tears of recognition: 'Because there have been several sudden and very painful losses in your life, things always seem uncertain for you. All your life you have been expecting the next catastrophe to strike'.

For this patient, cancer may be the most recent catastrophe, which acts as confirmation of the life script. For another patient, whose marriage broke down early and who has been unable to build another intimate relationship, a diagnosis of cancer may sound a death knell to the slender hope of finding a partner at midlife. Hence an early death feels less painful than having finally to relinquish the hope of sharing life with another person. For yet another patient, abused as a child, remaining in control of situations has been the paramount objective in adult life. The need to remain in control will prove very difficult in the context of treatment for cancer.

As this is a time-limited model, patients are kept to the central issue and are offered the correct amount of distance so that optimal autonomy is preserved. For many patients, termination begins at the sixth session, halfway through. The last three meetings are reserved for dealing with termination issues, and an intense termination often results from a telescoping of dynamic events within a brief period. Mann's model is suitable for patients presenting with loss issues; however those with very traumatic early histories and borderline pathology are poor candidates for this kind of brief work and can suffer psychological damage as a result. Although this model was not devised specifically for cancer patients, the emphasis on the patient's 'present and chronically endured pain' is an important feature.

A key counselling skill is an ability to formulate accurately the central issue and empathically communicate this to the patient. This ability is not easily acquired from reading alone, and counsellors need to be appropriately trained and supervised to use this model effectively. Brief psychodynamic therapy requires a high degree of skill, knowledge and experience. Short treatment does not imply easy treatment, even for an experienced therapist. The best preparation for doing brief therapy is a thorough knowledge of psychoanalytic theory and many years experience doing longer-term psychodynamic psychotherapy.

The Psychodynamic Formulation

At the heart of all brief psychodynamic therapies is the psychodynamic formulation, which is based on the problem and its history, the psychosocial history and the patient's behaviour during assessment interview(s). Sometimes events in the psychosocial history are fairly readily linked to the presenting problem. What follows are common patterns.

1. The dynamic formulation may relate an event in the past such as an early trauma to a current conflict; the present problem may be an unwitting repetition of an early experience, event, or interpersonal relationship

   - Mr J was repeatedly locked in cupboards as a child by his psychotic parents; under the radiotherapy machine, he is experiencing terrifying panic attacks.

2. Maladaptive behaviour has been unwittingly copied from parents or is a response to parental behaviour when the patient was a child

   - When Mrs C was a little girl, the only way she could gain attention from her mother was to throw noisy temper tantrums. When her cancer recurred, the tantrums reappeared and placed great stress on her family, who sought help.

3. An early conflict in the patient's childhood has endured into adult life

   - Ms D's little brother died when he was a few months old. She blamed herself for his death, as indeed did her distraught mother. Sarah chose a life of service in which her own needs were systematically disavowed. Diagnosed with a fast-growing cancer in her 30s, she is unable to receive any comfort or solace from family members. She is only 'collecting her fate', the punishment that has been waiting for her since she was a child.

4. There has been a developmental arrest leading to the current problem; certain stages of personality development have been incompletely negotiated, because of stress or trauma at the time

- Ms M's father died soon after her mother threw him out of the house for excessive drinking. After his death Ms M returned home in her early 20s to look after her depressed mother and never left to live her own life. In the cancer clinic, Ms M and her mother are a symbiotic unit. One cannot be seen without overwhelming interference from the other, and the resulting stress on medical staff has led to a referral for counselling.

5. Under the impact of early loss or failures of parenting, childhood solutions or 'survival kits' that were adaptive in the past have persisted into adult life and are now dysfunctional

- Mr A discovered that the most effective way of shutting out the 'madhouse' in which he lived as a boy was to retreat into books. His emotions were habitually suppressed and he took solace in intellectualization. This earned him two doctoral degrees and a high-paying job, but now that he has cancer he is finding it difficult to cope with his feelings.

6. Unconscious guilt is hindering the patient's adjustment in adult life; such guilt may stem from childhood abuse, for which patients blame themselves. A psychologist working with women in an obstetrics and gynaecology clinic highlights the importance of pathogenic beliefs from early abuse or trauma, especially beliefs involving guilt and punishment for perceived wrongdoing (Josephs 1996)

- Mother said, 'It would have been better if you had never been born'

- 'If I had gone downstairs with my little sister that morning, she wouldn't have put her nightdress onto the gas fire, and she wouldn't have died'

- 'This cancer came because of what happened to me in the street' [gang raped during the war, the patient blames herself].

7. Abused as children, in adult life the tables are turned, and someone else becomes the victim

   - Mr T's parents were ruthless in their treatment of him, allowing him to be physically and sexually abused by members of the extended family. When Mr T's wife developed a gynaecological cancer, he was irate that he was being deprived of sex. As he said to his counsellor, 'A woman is just a life support system for a vagina'.

In arriving at the psychodynamic formulation, special attention should be paid to the nature of the child's relationships with parents, the quality of adult relationships and any clues to transference reactions gleaned from the first hour. It is important that a careful assessment is made so that patients referred for brief psychodynamic therapy are able to use it effectively. Patients with longstanding psychiatric problems of a severe kind, childhood sexual abuse histories or sustained childhood trauma may need longer-term psychodynamic therapy from a specialist. Cancer patients who are also Holocaust survivors are a particularly vulnerable group (Baider *et al.* 1997).

Certain aspects of client-centred and cognitive-behavioural therapies described elsewhere in this book may be safely added to routine care with a modicum of training, whereas more intensive training and supervision are required of those who offer psychodynamic therapies to cancer patients.

9
The Client-centred Model

To give the patient the impression that you could spare him an hour and yet make him satisfied with five minutes is an invaluable gift. (Asher 1972)

Establishing a Counselling Relationship: General Principles

The first observation that needs to be made about the counselling relationship is the difference between this way of relating and friendship. Saying 'I'm like that too' or 'I felt like that once' is not a counselling response. The desire to share details of one's own experience with a patient is usually counterproductive and should be resisted. Counselling is a giving of one-way attention, and the helper's own feelings at the time are put to one side. It may be important that those feelings are attended to later in another setting, but not with the patient (Charles-Edwards 1983).

In a helpful booklet produced by BACUP, Buckman (1994) summarizes the basic principles in talking with people who have cancer:

- talking about distress helps relieve it
- a listener doesn't have to have the answers, just listening to the questions will help
- thoughts that a person tries to shut out will do harm

eventually; talking about fears and anxieties does not *create* them where they did not exist before.

There are some obvious obstacles to talking that are sometimes forgotten, even by those accustomed to a helping role. The person who is ill may want to talk, but helpers are too busy with other tasks. The listener may want to talk and the ill person does not, either because the feelings are too intense at that time, or no feelings come to mind. The ill person may want to talk but feels they ought not to, and the helper does not know how to encourage discussion. Or the ill person appears not to want to talk but really needs to, and the helper does not know what's best to do. A common fear is that intervening could make the situation worse. Timing is important: readiness to share feelings is the crucial factor.

Buckman advises sitting down, looking relaxed and signalling nonverbally that you're there to spend some time. A private room with no obstacles between you will help. Trying to keep your eyes on the same level as the person you're talking to also helps. This detail is often forgotten by doctors who are accustomed to standing over a patient, who may be either sitting in a chair or lying in a bed. Two feet or so between you and the other person is usually about right.

Find out whether the person who is ill wants to talk: 'Do you feel like talking?' is better than 'Tell me about your feelings', which is more directive. It is unhelpful to rehearse what you're going to say while the other person is still speaking and even more important not to interrupt or change the subject. When people stop talking, it is often because there is something painful or sensitive to discuss. It is important to wait at these times and not to rush. When there is something very difficult and you truly do not know what to say, a touch or an arm round a shoulder can sometimes be of greater value than words. From time to time it helps to check that you have not misunderstood. You might ask, 'How do you feel about that now?' or 'Can you help me understand what you mean a bit more?' There is often a temptation to give advice but this is almost always less helpful than staying with the difficult feelings. Some patients deal with the stress of illness with humour. If this is *their* coping style, it may help to share the joke.

However, attempting to cheer up the patient with a supply of jokes is usually for the helper's benefit, not the patient's.

At a time of illness, patients become exquisitely sensitive to the nonverbal messages sent by staff: does that person seem open, empathic and honest, or not? A patient described how she chose which doctor might be most willing to answer her questions (Souhami 1978):

> *I lay in bed and watched them as they went on the ward round and tried to decide which one would be most likely to tell me what I wanted to know. After I had made up my mind, I worked out exactly what I wanted him to tell me, then I told Sister which one I wanted to see and then I asked him my questions outright.*

It is sometimes debated whether good communication skills can be taught. Brewin (1977) points out that many of those who are best at it never analyse what they do, let alone write about it, and yet there is much that *can* be said, *can* be taught. Good communication with patients need not always take a lot of time. A few words of the right kind at the right time can make an enormous difference, and nonverbal communication can be vital (Brewin 1977):

> *Unspoken communication may have a greater impact than words. The patient may quickly decide, sometimes from little more than a smile or the firm touch of a hand, that the person speaking to him wants to help, knows how to and has at least some idea of how he or she feels. Even the busiest doctor should try to appear relaxed, unhurried and, above all, in a serious situation, not embarrassed or afraid and very willing to answer any questions.*

Similarly, nonverbal signs can indicate the wish to avoid discussion (Lichter 1987):

> *Tone of voice, demeanour and facial expression are ways in which staff may unconsciously tell patients that they do not wish to listen to them. At times attempts are [also] made to divert discussion into less difficult areas when patients or relatives try to talk about their worries. This can become such an automatic response that carers do not realize they are doing it.*

Lack of time can be a barrier. Gifted doctors make every patient feel worthwhile and deserving of attention. They do not say, 'There are nine other patients on this ward and I have to get to them now'. The sensitive general practitioner does the same thing with the seven-minute consultation, being fully present and listening as if there were all the time in the world for that person during those few minutes. There is not unlimited time, of course, but the patient *feels* as if there is and feels cared for and heard.

A very helpful list of objectives within the initial medical consultation has been assembled (Crisp 1986), incorporating principles of good psychological care:

- create the right atmosphere in terms of physical ambience, personal sensitivity, empathy and concern

- identify and share with the patient the purposes of the interview

- listen attentively and receptively, enabling the patient to volunteer personal information and to feel involved in his or her own care

- pursue fully the complaint and its history with its psychological, social and personal aspects

- understand and use nonverbal communication

- redirect the patient where necessary without disturbing the flow of the interview

- deploy open-ended questions and closed questions appropriately in pursuit of precision, clarification of inconsistencies and a comprehensive understanding of the problem

- tolerate emotionally disturbing things that the patient might say

- use a style that is appropriate to each patient at each stage of the interview

- avoid jargon and explain the meaning of medical terms

- define and communicate, when appropriate, underlying meanings that reveal themselves as the interview proceeds

- minimize defensiveness by an accepting nonverbal manner

- recognize when an interview is failing and make appropriate adjustments

- answer questions clearly and accurately

- remember what has been said

- enable the patient to understand your recommendations and the effects of accepting or rejecting them

- formulate and summarize well for the record.

Those who wish to read in more detail about the initial medical consultation might consult Eric Cassell's *Talking With Patients*, volume 2 (1985), an excellent text on the medical interview, with its opening question, 'Tell me the story of this illness, please'. Cassell describes how to ask questions about the body, take a personal history, explore the personal meaning of the illness to the patient and use information as a therapeutic tool. In *The Healer's Art* (1976), Cassell explores in more general terms the nature of the doctor–patient relationship. He stresses the need for health workers to understand the meaning of the illness *to this particular patient at this particular time*. 'The major complaint people have about their doctors is that they don't listen. Listening means hearing not only what the symptoms are but what they mean to the patient.'

According to Cassell, the doctor's explanation has three parts: what the trouble is, what it means in body terms and what it means in person terms. For the patient the most important bit may be a fourth part: 'the causal term, the "why" part of the sentence, which for some patients is the most important because it helps fix the "blame" for the condition. Patients want to know if the cause of their illness is heredity or overwork, but the one seemingly unacceptable causal term is fate'. For the cancer patient, the causal term may be the most important part of the medical sentence. 'The four parts of the medical sentence are always hanging in the air, so to speak. If the physician fails to fill in the missing information, the patient will obtain it elsewhere' (Cassell 1976).

Another resource is Brian Bird's *Talking With Patients* (1973). Success will be enhanced if the helper 'acts like a cheerful human being sincerely interested in another human being....

Quizzing, grilling and the third degree have no place at all in talking with patients'. Bird suggests that the doctor try to keep conversation going during the physical examination because sometimes some of the most helpful revelations pop out in a casual way during that time. It is also important to listen for connections between the bits of information being offered (Bird 1973).

> For example, asked how long his symptoms had been present, a patient said: 'Let's see, my mother died two months ago. This started a week later, so it's almost two months'. The doctor was silent a moment, then asked, 'What is your occupation?' Why the doctor did not follow up the obvious relationship between onset of the patient's symptoms and the death of the mother was most likely due to some anxiety of his own ... Be particularly interested in the sequence of events, the order in which things took place ... Use open-ended questions such as 'And then?'; 'And before that, what?' ... Don't be in a hurry. A patient's slowness or reluctance is in itself an informative fact. Give patients time to warm up, and if time runs out, let them come back. Sometimes a second session is remarkably different from an initial one.

The First Counselling Session

When the primary aim of a first meeting is to counsel, the goal should be to help the patient to disclose feelings. This is the opposite of the usual structured medical history-taking process, where the aim is to make a diagnosis and prescribe treatment. Counselling is not a process of information giving, rather the aim is to make the person as comfortable as possible so they feel able to talk. Attributes that facilitate this process have been described by Rogers (1957) and include empathy, genuineness and an unconditional positive regard for the patient.

The communication skills needed in the professional–patient encounter generally involve the following tasks.

Beginning the encounter. Putting the other at ease, establishing an appropriate working relationship, clarifying goals and ascertaining what the patient already knows are all initial steps.

Questioning. Probing and prompting uses open-ended questions, for example, 'Can you tell me a bit more about that?'

When questions are used, it is important to express them clearly and to avoid an aggressive stance.

Listening. Looking at the patient is a crucial element and all listening needs to be supported with appropriate nonverbal cues, in other words the need to look as if what is being heard is of interest to the listener. Listening effectively also involves accepting feelings and acknowledging them to the person telling the story.

Explaining. It is vital to consider the speed and complexity of any explanation being offered to the patient and to consider whether the language being used is appropriate. Jargon can be a barrier to patients communicating further. It is helpful to allow some pauses when giving an explanation as this gives the patient time to take in what is being said. Feedback questions can be vital, for example 'Does what I say make sense?', 'Did I say that too quickly for you?', 'Would you like me to go through that again?' When giving an explanation it is important to check for verbal or nonverbal cues given by patients signifying they have not understood.

Acknowledging. This involves the acceptance of the patient's emotional responses: 'Uh huh', 'Yes' or 'Right'. The amount and variety of this reinforcing is timed to encourage further disclosure.

Reflecting feelings. This involves using technigues to open up feelings and bring them out into the dialogue, for example, 'It sounds like you're pretty fed up at the moment', 'That seems like an upsetting thing for you', or 'So you're feeling very scared at the moment'. It is a prerequisite of the reflective technique that the feelings be identified in order that they can be reflected. This is not to say that it is necessary to always be accurate at first about the feeling being expressed but it is important to convey you are trying to understand what that feeling may be: 'So it's not that your feeling scared but you're a bit apprehensive, perhaps?'

Paraphrasing. This can be done in such a way as to summarize for the purpose of clarification, for example, 'Let me just see if I have understood...' or 'So what you are saying is...'.

Variation. The demonstration of interest and enthusiasm can be achieved by body language and by vocal changes.

Sustaining. It is important to allow and facilitate the expression of strong feelings, understand the reasons for those feelings and, in some instances, redirect them into a more helpful mode.

Closure. Ending any encounter with a patient requires some summarizing of the main points that have been covered by both patient and the counsellor. At this point it is useful to check that the patient's intentions or expectations have been met. This is also the point at which to draw a link between what has happened in the consultation and any future action to be taken.

The first meeting involves getting to know the patient and forming a picture of what sort of person they are. It also involves some evaluation of how they are coping as this can influence in an important way how any subsequent encounters proceed. The first meeting can not only involve learning about the patient and making a formulation but it can also have therapeutic benefit in its own right. In the process of telling their story, some worries may be disclosed and this is part of what counselling offers. However, counselling can also go beyond ventilation of emotions. Even the initial counselling session can be used to introduce the notion of change. It is not enough simply to encourage ventilation, because coping also involves looking at what needs to be changed in order to make life less distressing. Therefore, counselling can also involve some discussion of how it may be possible to alter things so that it becomes easier to cope with cancer and to develop a positive and more optimistic approach to life. A first step may be to encourage patients to define their priorities, as in the case of Miss M.

Miss M came for counselling following her cancer treatment. Like many patients, her concern was about whether the disease would return. However, these worries had become overwhelming to the point that she was unable to engage in her normal activities

continued

continued

because of a feeling of helplessness. Initially, much of the time was spent simply talking about these worries, which she felt unable to discuss with those who were close to her because she felt they would not understand why she was so worried and because it would simply cause them to become upset and over-protective towards her. In this discussion it became apparent that her main agenda revolved around gaining some enjoyment from life and re-establishing her plans for her job. With help, she was able to focus on methods for achieving these aims. This involved her using the discussion as a sounding board rather than her being offered advice.

Her main priority became to recommence classes in drama and push forward on plans she had to pass a professional examination. This allowed her to confirm her future priorities and make practical plans aimed at achieving these goals. The worries about the disease receded as she focused her attention and energies on the need to achieve these priorities. Engaging in the practical steps needed to achieve her priorities had further benefits as this provided evidence that she was able to carry on without feeling overwhelmed by disease-related worries. The activities themselves served as an additional distraction bringing her some further relief.

Helpers' Resistances to Listening to Feelings

Although one of the principal aims of counselling is the ventilation of feelings, many helpers consciously or unconsciously discourage people from expressing negative emotions. Sometimes this avoidance is rooted in a personal wish to stay away from upsetting issues. At other times it is cloaked under the excuse, 'I don't have time to talk about these things with patients', or 'I haven't been trained to do this'. Many distressing feelings are commonly experienced by cancer patients. Shame and humiliation are two very unpleasant feelings that patients are likely to experience at some time during the course of the illness (Lazare 1987):

Patients are at high risk for experiencing shame and humiliation in any medical encounter. This is because they commonly perceive diseases as defects, inadequacies, or short-comings, while the visit to the hospital and the doctor's office requires physical and psychological exposure. Patients respond to the suffering of shame and humiliation by avoiding the physician, withholding information, complaining and suing.

'Dying with dignity' is often about worry concerning such things as excessive water retention, emaciation, deformity, mutilation, incontinence and the need to use a bedpan. Once in the consulting room, patients are asked to reveal personal information (often about their weaknesses), expose their bodies for examination, place themselves in undignified postures and accept the handling of their bodies by strangers, including the introduction of fingers or instruments into private parts of the body. The most common patient reaction to shame is to become quiet and withdrawn. Unfortunately some doctors deliberately shame their patients, for example, 'How do you expect me to help you when you continue to smoke?' Patients who have been on the receiving end of this approach will usually change their doctor if they are able to do so. The doctor can help the patient by assuring privacy, showing empathy for the patient's plight and acknowledging shame and humiliation by saying something like, 'It is not easy to come and see a doctor about this; it was wise of you to come today'.

Some doctors use the defence of speaking in jargon, which maintains their position of power and ensures that patients don't understand. Others accomplish the same result by being so visibly rushed that patients do not dare to speak to them. As one patient put it, 'They don't stand still long enough for you to draw a bead on 'em ... And when they tell you something you very often don't understand it because it is said in such fancy language that it leaves a lot to your imagination' (Skipper 1965).

In one study, medical students found it difficult to talk with patients about sexual and marital problems, and they were concerned about what they should say if the patient asked, 'Am I dying?' They were uncertain whether doctors should be honest with patients and whether a doctor should ever admit to having made a mistake. What was the doctor to say if a patient has read her general practitioner's letter and the patient disagrees with the diagnosis? How should the doctor deal with patients who have had their condition explained twice but who still ask about it, and how should the doctor behave with a patient who is rejecting, angry or hostile? This is an interesting list of concerns, including the basic life issues of caring for others, honesty, sex, aggression and death. In the role-play sessions that were offered, one student said, 'We are frightened that we may show part of ourselves' (MacNamara 1974). This profoundly revealing remark brings to mind the distinction in health care between the **instrumental** and **expressive** functions. Doctors and nurses have many instrumental functions: taking a history, giving information, making diagnoses, writing prescriptions, ordering treatments, referring to colleagues and carrying out medical, surgical or nursing procedures. In the course of these activities, they may be able to conceal successfully their personal weaknesses and concerns beneath the acquired skills.

However, the counselling side of the work *requires* that helpers reveal, or express, aspects of themselves, since the principal tool of counselling is the counsellor's self. And if there are in the helper, as there very often are, conflicts around caring for others, honesty, sexual intimacy, anger, aggression and death, they *will* show. This may be one of the reasons some helpers do what they can to stay away from patients' strong feelings. To be a good counsellor requires an openness to one's own strong feelings. Otherwise our defences and blind spots will get in the way of looking after other people. Some helpers have developed defences against feelings that are so ingrained they are almost automatic. Maguire (1985) speaks of some of these as distancing tactics. One common one is changing the subject. False reassurance is another (Shields 1984).

> Too many times cliché phrases such as 'You should be strong at times like this', 'Don't cry, she will think you are weak', 'Try to be cheerful' or 'Don't get angry' are offered as well-meaning advice. The patient attempts to abide by these moral imperatives, all of which demand a distortion of true feelings.

Patients who do not want Counselling

Not every cancer patient needs or wants counselling. Many are only temporarily distressed and adapt well in the long term. When a counselling programme was offered to cancer patients in an American hospital, Worden and Weisman (1980) found a number of patients did not want help. 'Hard' refusers were firmly inaccessible from the outset. They became more and more recalcitrant, truculent and even suspicious as the interviewer explained the programme. By contrast, 'soft' refusers shunned the interviewer more in sorrow than in anger. The authors point out that by rejecting help, refusers are no less at risk. Trouble may still await the patient who refuses counselling. Hard refusers may be a lost cause while soft refusers may become more amenable to counselling later. In a study of 300 breast cancer patients in the Midlands, 80 patients declined to be interviewed preoperatively when approached in hospital, but two-thirds of them agreed to be followed up one year after the operation. Those who declined were older, less worried overall one year after surgery and used less fighting spirit and anxious preoccupation at one year than did patients in the experimental groups (Burton and Parker 1995). They generally seemed to have adjusted philosophically to their lot, and they did not wish to speak to anyone about their feelings. Such preferences on the part of patients should always be respected.

Talking with People about their Feelings: A Practical Guide

Talking with patients about their feelings need not be a lengthy, time-consuming activity. Even a sentence or two that accurately reflects the feeling being expressed can be helpful. The aim of this approach is to help the other person feel heard at the feeling level. These skills can be learned, but to be effective they require a desire to hear what the other person wants to say. People can tell if we are using a technique and do not really want to listen. Talking with people about their feelings requires three basic attitudes (Rogers 1951):

- empathy, the ability to sense the other person's world of felt meanings as if they were our own, but without ever losing the 'as if' quality

- unconditional positive regard, a positive, warm, accepting response to the other, regardless of how difficult their behaviour may be at the moment; the assumption that behind the difficult behaviour is a feeling, suffering person

• openness to feelings, communicating to the other person that whatever the feeling is we can accept it; any feeling can be talked about.

Empathic listening means immersing yourself in the world of the other, allowing yourself to resonate to both spoken and unspoken messages and being aware of your own feelings and associations as you listen. Patients should be encouraged to explore, to pursue their own leads and to make their own discoveries. As listeners, we should attend silently until we feel we have a reasonable understanding of what the other person is trying to communicate. It is a useful discipline to listen for the theme or themes of the hour, resisting the temptation to be clever or brilliant and being tentative in communications to the other.

It is important to be alert to occasions when the patient may hear a communication as a criticism or rebuke. It can be helpful to step back a moment and ask yourself silently, 'I wonder how the patient experienced what I just said'. If something unhelpful has been said, it is best to apologize, for example, 'I may have been unhelpful to you when I said such-and-such'. If in doubt, examine what you are about to say and ask yourself, 'Is this in the patient's best interest or mine?' (Strupp and Binder 1984; Casement 1985).

The nonverbal component to the communication of empathy, unconditional positive regard and openness to feelings is particularly important. It is difficult to describe in words and is probably best learned through videotape feedback on our performance. Other people can tell whether we seem to be empathic, whether we like them or not and whether certain feelings can be discussed. They probably could not tell us exactly how they know these things, but when patients are ill and feeling vulnerable, they often very rapidly assess those around them in precisely these terms.

Gordon (1970) identified 12 types of communication, 'the typical twelve', that are best avoided when counselling.

1. Commanding, telling the other person what to do: 'Don't speak to staff that way!'
2. Warning, telling the other person what will happen if they persist in this behaviour: 'If you carry on ringing that bell for the nurse, you'll be sorry'.
3. Preaching, telling people what they ought to do: 'You shouldn't behave like that when people are trying to help you'.
4. Giving solutions, trying to solve the other person's problem for them: 'I suggest you speak to your children about that'.
5. Lecturing, trying to influence the other with facts, logic or your own opinions: 'If you'll just cooperate with the treatment, things will go much better'.
6. Judging, making a negative judgment: 'I'm afraid you're not thinking very clearly'.
7. Praising, offering a positive evaluation or judgment: 'I don't think it looks that bad' (when the other person feels it looks terrible).
8. Name-calling, making someone feel put down or foolish: 'Now look here, smart aleck'.
9. Interpreting, analysing why people are doing what they're doing, telling them you have them figured out: 'You're thinking this because you are a very suspicious sort of person'.
10. Reassuring, an effort to make the person feel better, when there is no guarantee that things will go well: 'Everything is going to turn out all right, my dear, don't worry'.
11. Questioning, searching for more information in order to help you solve the problem: 'When was the first time you felt this way?'
12. Distracting, pushing the problem aside: 'Aren't those flowers beautiful!'

The alternative to the 12 responses is listening for the feeling and reflecting that feeling back in an accepting manner. You want to communicate that whatever the feeling is, you would like to hear more about it. Listening in this way carries with it the risk that you might be affected emotionally by what you hear. Because of this risk, you may close off this kind of conversation with a defence mechanism such as one of the typical twelve. Many of the typical twelve have a useful place in certain circumstances; however any one of them can be used by the counsellor defensively.

Inviting more communication

Invitations for the other person to say more can be made in several ways:

- silence
- a nonverbal attending attitude: good eye contact and an open body posture
- 'Um hm', 'Uh huh', 'Ah', 'Oh', 'Right', 'Yes', 'I see'
- 'It sounds like you have strong feelings about that'
- 'It sounds like this is very hard for you'
- 'Could you say a bit more about that?'

It is important, when you use encouragements like this, to keep the door open and respond to whatever the feeling is that the other person would like to share.

Reflecting the feeling that the other person is communicating

When you are first learning the skills involved in communicating back the feelings you are hearing, model responses such as the following, in which the feeling is named using a single word, may help:

- It *sounds like* you're feeling ...
- So you're feeling *sort of* ...
- So there's a feeling of ...

It is helpful to make your response tentative, so the other person can either accept your comment or go on to say that the feeling is something else. It is alright to pick up the wrong feeling, and you *will* pick up the wrong feeling often, as long as it is also alright for the other person to say, 'No, it's not that, it's more this other thing'. Then they will tell you what it is, and you can go on from there. Do not worry excessively about reflecting the wrong feeling back to the other person, initially. If your reflection is made tentatively, you are letting them know that, whatever the feeling is, you would like to hear more about it. Sometimes you may have picked up the feeling accurately but they do not want to face that with you yet. You may be able to return to it later on. They are more likely to come back to it if you make your first response tentative.

Some common feelings

Feelings are best reflected back to the other person as a single word or a very brief phrase. There are words that are typically used in association with certain types of feeling, for example:

- depressive feelings: low, worthless, miserable, guilty, hopeless, helpless, bleak
- angry feelings: betrayed, cheated, frustrated, furious
- frightened feelings: apprehensive, overwhelmed, afraid, terrified, scared stiff, upset (the last of which can be a euphemism for almost any negative feeling)
- positive feelings: at peace, excited, comforted, confident, hopeful
- neutral feelings: cautious, uncertain, confused, self-conscious, stuck, mixed up, distant, not bothered, surprised.

Those feelings we find most difficult to describe in ourselves may well be the feelings we find hardest to explore with other people. When these feelings come up in conversation, we may use one of the typical twelve to defend ourselves against getting too closely in touch with our own discomfort.

Sequences of feelings

Very often it is not only one feeling that is being expressed. Sequences of feelings can be especially useful to explore, especially when those sequences occur as part of a recurring pattern.

- Every time *anger* is experienced, it is followed by a feeling of *guilt*: 'I was absolutely furious with him and we had a terrific row. Then I went to my room and cried because I felt so bad about it'.

- The first feeling may be *hurt*, then *anger* and then *guilt*: 'First I was just overwhelmed by the hurt. Then I felt furious. And now I'm beginning to wonder what I did to make it happen'.

- As the prospect of intimacy arises, the patient is flooded first with feelings of *need*, then *fear*: 'I'd begun to realize how much I wanted to be with her. Then I got terrified. She took my hand and I recoiled'.

- In attempting to *cope* with the illness alone, others may be *devalued*: 'She's not really that important – I don't need her anyway'.

- At a time of loss, *helplessness* may be followed by feelings of *worthlessness*, intense *fear*, *sadness* and *emptiness*: 'I am alone now. Things will never get better. Without him, I am worthless and I will fall apart. I feel so sad and empty all the time, and the future is terrifying. There is no future for me'.

- After the loss of someone who had hurt, controlled and deprived a person, there may be feelings of *guilt*, *anger* and *sadness*: 'She was incapable of being an adequate mother to me. I can never forgive her for what she did, but now I think that somehow I caused her death. And at the same time she had such a tragic life. It all feels very sad'.

Key interpersonal issues

Another useful way of listening for themes is in terms of key interpersonal issues, such as the following.

Intimacy

- excessive need for intimacy or denial of need for intimacy
- fear that intimacy will result in abandonment
- incapacity for intimacy owing to excessive preoccupation with self
- incapacity to maintain an intimate relationship over a period of time
- capacity for intimacy overwhelmed by aggressive impulses
- feeling undeserving of an intimate relationship
- choosing a partner who is incapable of intimacy.

Control

- overuse of control, lack of control or inconsistency in control
- strong need to control others as well as the self
- choice of partner with excessive control or poor control.

Dependency

- denial or exaggeration of dependent needs
- unable to make self vulnerable for fear of abandonment
- guilt and shame about dependency
- narcissistic rage when dependent needs go unmet
- inability to choose appropriate persons on whom to depend.

Trust

- inability to trust others or too trusting of others, too 'naive'
- feeling that the world is an unsafe place
- fear that trusting others will result in betrayal
- choice of untrustworthy partners.

Anger

- inability to express anger or fear of aggression towards others when angry
- anger expressed in a violent and uncontrollable fashion
- anger always followed by a feeling of guilt or fear
- fear of retaliation from those with whom one has been angry
- choice of partners who cannot express anger or deal with anger in others
- choice of partners who cannot control anger.

Sexuality

- inhibition of sexual desire, denial of sexual needs
- inability to let go and experience orgasm
- incapable of controlling sexual impulses: sexual acting out
- infiltration of sexual impulses with aggression
- inability to integrate sexuality with intimacy (one partner for love, another for sex)
- inability to become sexually excited with spouse, only with a lover
- self or partner becomes 'all bad' after a sexual encounter
- sexual partner is inappropriately idealized, 'put on a pedestal'
- inability to see sexual partner as a whole person
- choice of inappropriate sexual partners.

Self-disclosure

- unable to talk about feelings
- too ready to self-disclose and to inappropriate people
- self-disclosure is not accompanied by insight or under-standing

- to say nothing is safer (passive–aggressive response)
- choice of partner who is unable to talk about feelings.

Boundaries

- no boundaries between people: people 'flow into' one another
- no respect for existing boundaries between people
- setting up or seeking situations that threaten or violate boundaries
- too rigid reliance on boundaries to defend against intimacy
- choice of partner who has either inadequate or too rigid boundary control

Rejection

- incapable of intimacy because terrified of rejection
- does the rejecting first, before the other can do it (pre-emptive strike)
- rejects others contemptuously, as inferior
- responds to rejection with helplessness and hopelessness
- sees self as rejected, unloved and worthless
- misperceives commonplace events as rejection
- choice of rejecting partner.

Separation

- incapable of separating from parents
- responds to separation with feelings of helplessness and hopelessness
- defends against pain of separation by 'feeling nothing'
- responds to separation with narcissistic rage reaction
- responds to separation with feelings of guilt

- responds to separation with emptiness or inner desolation
- unable to separate from destructive or abusing partner
- choice of dependent partner to defend against prospect of separation

The use of metaphors

In speaking about their problems, patients will sometimes use vivid metaphors that can be used to understand life themes. For example:

A woman describes herself as walking a tightrope, high above the rest of the world. People below are going about their business and developing relationships. Out of her fear of intimacy, and because of two traumatic losses in the past, she is living in a kind of splendid isolation high above the fray, where her consuming preoccupation is keeping herself from falling off the tightrope. It became possible to talk about people below inviting her to come down.

A man describes how during the potato famine, farm tenants were evicted to spend the winter in a hole in the ground. Men, pregnant women, babies and the aged went to live in these pits with a roof of branches and turf, where few survived. Water poured through the roofs and illness and death quickly followed. The atmosphere was one of acute deprivation, loss of loved ones, lack of food and warmth and waiting for death. This metaphor was a picture of how this man viewed life.

Common problems in active listening

- If an issue has been identified and the other person doesn't want to talk about it: 'It sounds like you don't want to talk about that right now'. If the answer is no, this should be respected. Your saying, 'right now' leaves the door open to talk about it later, if they wish.

- If they do seem to want to talk but are having difficulty expressing feelings: 'It seems that this is very difficult to discuss', or 'All of this sounds very painful and upsetting and hard to talk about'.

- Sometimes people break down and cry, in which case a tissue box on the table is helpful and, after an appropriate interval, to say something like: 'Perhaps you've been needing to let go of these feelings for awhile'. If the person apologizes for crying, you might say: 'You don't need to apologize for crying, crying is OK in here'.

- Sometimes people get very angry at us but may feel they do not have permission to express it: 'You seemed very angry at me when I gave you bad news', or 'So there's a lot of anger in you about the recurrence'.

- Sometimes feelings are being expressed quite freely up to some point, and then there is a block. You can still reflect the feeling of being blocked: 'It seemed like it was easy for you to talk about this until you got on to the topic of your relationship with your mother. Then it became very difficult for you to go on'. Sometimes just focusing on the block, or naming the 'something' that is blocking by, as it were, pointing to 'it', can release it.

- Sometimes it can be helpful, if you are not sure what the feeling is, to repeat the last few words, or a short phrase from what the other person has said: 'So this is a "brand new experience"'. This technique, however, can be over-used and should be employed with caution.

Reflecting feelings: coping styles

Coping styles in dealing with cancer were discussed in Chapter 3. If we are using a client-centred or Rogerian approach, we do not attempt to alter the patient's coping style but reflect back to the patient what we have heard:

- denial: 'So you're not sure you actually have cancer'
- fighting spirit: 'It sounds like you're going to fight this'

- stoic acceptance: 'So this is something you have decided to put up with and accept'
- helplessness: 'So the whole idea of this illness makes you feel hopeless and depressed'
- anxious preoccupation: 'You seem to be spending a lot of time looking for lumps and worrying about recurrence'.

Such a technique allows the patient to say more about the coping style that has been adopted and to explore the underlying feelings further. This nondirective approach is different from the cognitive–behavioural model described in Chapter 10 and may be more suitable for certain patients.

How reflecting feelings works therapeutically

When we have accurately reflected a feeling, the intervention is successful when the patient says, 'That's right, *and another thing is...*' There is always more than one feeling about a situation, and the therapeutic task is to explore as many of these feelings as possible (Gendlin 1962). We are on the right track when the discussion moves from one feeling to another: 'So you feel very angry, but another part of you feels ashamed'. When people are able to express accurately in words for the first time how they are feeling, at that moment they are no longer that way. In the act of sharing the feeling with another person, the feeling has already changed. Only certain words will fit exactly the way a person feels at one time. When the right words are found, that discovery is accompanied by the feeling, 'That's exactly right', and when the feeling has become capable of being named, it has already changed and may lead to the discovery of other, related feelings: 'That's exactly right, and the other thing is...' This increased access to the range of feelings facilitates decision-making and the resolution of crises.

Even when the feeling is not clear and no adequate words can be found, one can point to the unclear feeling as a 'that', or 'that feeling, whatever it is'. The expression, '...or something like that' can be very useful. It is as if one is pointing to a part of the patient's inner life; it may as yet have no name, but it can be identified as an 'over there', or 'that block I can't get past'. The process can then move on from there (Gendlin 1967).

Client-centred counselling with cancer patients

The reflection-of-feelings technique can be taught to medical and surgical staff, general practitioners, nurses, social workers, psychologists, liaison psychiatrists and others in allied fields who have not had a training in psychotherapy. Study days and workshops can be organized using written materials, demonstrations, videotaped exercises and role plays. Recent research suggests that these skills can be learned by surgical staff, and that even brief interventions of 30 minutes' duration can show benefits in psychological adjustment a year postsurgery in breast cancer patients (Burton and Parker 1995).

10
The Cognitive–Behavioural Model

The inclusion of psychological therapies within oncology should bring closer the ideal to which medicine pays lip service but which is rarely achieved, namely the treatment of the whole person. (Greer 1991)

A substantial minority of people often need further counselling and psychological support beyond what is offered in a routine way to cancer patients, and that help may need to be more structured in order to foster changes in how people cope with worries and concerns. What is described below is a brief psychological intervention designed specifically for cancer patients and their families. Theoretically this approach is based on cognitive–behavioural therapy as described by Beck (1976) and Meichenbaum (1977) and developed by Moorey and Greer (1989).

The psychodynamic life narrative in Chapter 8 focuses on the life setting of illness and the meaning of cancer at a particular time in a person's life. The Rogerian approach described in Chapter 9 is based on a here-and-now, reflection-of-feelings model. Taken together, the psychodynamic and Rogerian models may be sufficient to help many patients. Others may require a more structured or directive approach, especially if they are suffering from acute anxiety or severe depression.

The cognitive–behavioural model is based on the idea that thoughts contribute in an important way to how we feel. In this respect, thinking is causal: changing the way we think about something may change the way we feel. This is the 'cognitive' in cognitive therapy. Whether or not we agree with this model of human emotion is, however, less important than the techniques that are used to achieve changes in how people feel. In the model we present in this chapter, the techniques of cognitive-behavioural therapy have been adapted for use with cancer patients.

Ventilation of Emotions

The first step in encouraging positive thinking is common to most counselling methods and involves encouraging people to ventilate their concerns and problems. The general steps taken to facilitate ventilation have been described in Chapter 9 and draw on the Rogerian concepts of empathy, genuineness and unconditional positive regard. Ventilation of worries can be helped along if you show that you understand the medical background and events. If it is not possible to gain access to patients' medical notes then it is important to ask if they would like to recount what has happened. Sometimes it is helpful to ask them to do this anyway. Often this means asking them to go back to events at the time of their diagnosis. This process can be immensely revealing and should never be hurried as it allows them to tell you their story. From this, a host of things can be learned. If the patient is feeling angry it may be because they consider that their general practitioner was slow in referring them to a specialist. If they feel depressed it may be because of what they understand, or fail to understand, about their prognosis. If they feel anxious it may be because they are awaiting the results of a medical test.

This process of emotional ventilation will also clarify how the patient or family member has been trying to cope with perceived difficulties. It will give insight into the person telling the story. The process of ventilation is not necessarily fully achieved in a first meeting but is likely to continue throughout the relationship with the patient. However, it is important that some ventilation is allowed before offering patients a more structured approach to dealing with their problems. This model shares with other approaches the need to encourage patients to ventilate and share their worries. However, from this point it diverges and takes a more specific path. It is a short-term intervention lasting usually between four and eight sessions; it is problem-oriented and driven by patients' agendas; it is collaborative and educational in that the patient is taught coping strategies; it makes use of homework assignments; and it forms the basis for a self-help programme.

Initially the aims are to help patients gain relief from their emotional symptoms, to look at how they might live an ordinary life, to encourage the expression of feelings and to teach the cognitive model. In the beginning it can help patients if it is emphasized that the feelings they have are understandable and not unusual given the problems they are facing. It is also appropriate early on to introduce the basic plan for therapy – sometimes referred to as the treatment contract – by giving a brief outline of what is offered and what time commitment it involves.

As part of the process of introducing the model and 'normalizing' negative feelings, a short leaflet that patients can take home can be helpful. Written materials can form the basis of a self-help programme, with patients going back to the leaflets in future, if necessary, to remind themselves of the coping methods they can use. It is also helpful because anxious people find it difficult to take everything in and may forget quite a lot of what has been discussed in the session; the leaflets, therefore, act as a memory aid. The introduction of written materials provides an opportunity to clarify that any benefit is more likely to come about as a result of the changes patients are able to make in their day-to-day behaviours rather than from within the sessions themselves; that the sessions can serve as a forum for discussion of progress or lack of progress in coping; and that they can use the written materials to remind themselves of how to plan changes as part of a self-help strategy.

Behavioural Techniques

Behavioural techniques can be helpful initially because they often bring quite rapid symptom relief in terms of depression and anxiety. One of the most useful ways of helping patients plan how they can live an ordinary life is through the use of **activity scheduling**. Making a list of daily activities helps people to focus on the structure of their day, examines the nature and number of the activites they engage in and looks at how much pleasure and sense of control they are able to achieve within those activites. A useful didactic tool involves them in keeping a simple timetable of their activities, which they first complete as a baseline. This can be used for inpatients and outpatients, although the limitations of the hospital stay needs to be taken into account in planning activities with inpatients.

What frequently happens when people are diagnosed with cancer is that their normal daily activities are seriously disrupted. Things that were part of the usual structure of their life get pushed aside by medical events and by thoughts about cancer. Also physical symptoms from both the disease and the medical treatment impinge on the person's ability to undertake their usual activities and to gain enjoyment from them. Patients who become depressed in these circumstances are often spending substantial parts of their day doing very little, thus giving them plenty of time to ruminate about their problems and rehearse any worries thoroughly.

Activity scheduling is a process of negotiation that begins by looking at these timetables and asking things such as:

What did you used to do at these times?

Why do you feel unable to do these things at the moment? (Asked only if they are outpatients or there is no indication of physical symptoms that might prevent them engaging in their normal activities.)

Can you think of any things that you would like to do? (Within any limitations imposed by symptoms or the confines of hospital.)

What have you given up doing that you used to enjoy?

How can you get back to doing your normal activites within the constraints of your treatment or any physical symptoms you have at present?

What goals would you like to set so you can gradually shift back to a normal life?

What *is* normal life for you?

Are there perhaps some new things you want to try to begin?

Patients are then asked to rate specific activities in terms of how much pleasure it gives them and how much of a sense of mastery it provides. Then they can be encouraged to explore methods for increasing those things that give them a greater sense of pleasure and control. This is an important aim because it helps to give back some of the sense of being in control of one's life that the disease has taken away. Patients can keep a record of the number of activities they undertake and the pleasure or control it provides. This can then be compared with the baseline as a way of emphasizing that progress is occurring. The latter may be important because often if there has been a bad day, this serves to plunge them back into thinking they are back to square one.

Spouse or Partner as Co-therapist

The patient's partner can often be an important ally in the therapeutic process. First, however, it is important to ascertain how much distress the partner is experiencing and, where appropriate, address these problems either on an individual basis or as a couple. The notion of the partner as co-therapist is not difficult to get across to patients. One can explain that if the patient is to plan changes to the pattern of their day through activity scheduling, it is helpful to have someone there to encourage this and increase their motivation at a time when it may be at a low ebb. The best person to do this is the person with whom the patient shares their life. Together with the couple, it is possible to negotiate the implementation of changes to the daily routine through activity scheduling. Most people, regardless of whether or not they are psychologically minded, can make use of this approach and it often brings quite rapid relief of distress. This approach can help to lift feelings of depression in those whose symptoms are of mild to moderate intensity and can also help in the relief of anxiety. Encouragement and identification of specific aims or activities helps the process so that a clear structure is in place that the patient can attempt to follow.

The relief of symptoms seems to be achieved in several ways. First, the notion that life can be normal is encouraging.

It is also important that people begin to plan and structure what they do. Planning ahead often goes completely out the window at the time of diagnosis or during periods of crisis. Activity scheduling encourages people back to something we all do every day, which is to plan ahead, either short term or long term; it reaffirms that despite cancer life can go on, no matter how long or short. It also encourages people to take control of things through planning. The involvement in activities themselves can be beneficial either because they give pleasure or simply because they are distracting. Some people have a special need to engage their thoughts in something other than cancer. When this effort is fully successful it also demonstrates that it is possible not to feel overwhelmed by cancer all of the time.

At the very least this approach can provide patients with brief periods of respite from the distress they feel. All of this can be explained to the patient and their partner, and the important role the partner can play is emphasized. Although this places some burden of responsibility on the partner it can be therapeutic for those partners who are themselves distressed; it acts by focusing their attention on an active method by which they can help the patient and themselves to put their lives back together again after the crisis of cancer has hit them.

A note of caution is needed. Not all partners welcome this responsibility. Some can cope only by cutting themselves off and avoiding the emotional impact of what is happening. In these circumstances, they are not happy to engage in a dialogue that revolves around the issues of cancer. Sometimes the counsellor has to take on single-handedly the role of encouraging patients to resume their normal activities. This approach can also be used to help spouses or partners who are failing to cope but are willing to discuss new methods for coping.

Cognitive Techniques

Some of the anxiety and depression experienced by people who continue to fail to cope with having cancer can be attributed to their thinking processes. Often people feel low-spirited and depressed because they have very negative thoughts about themselves, the disease and the future: 'I'm useless', 'I'll never get better', 'I'll never be able to do any of the things I used to'. Such thinking tends to reduce the motivation to do anything; patients become locked into a vicious circle where they are unable to motivate themselves to do things and then feel worse because this reinforces their sense of uselessness. These negative thoughts often spring to mind automatically, without much awareness and with little effort to control them. Sometimes these negative thoughts become quite distorted and do not represent reality. Such thoughts, however, may seem quite plausible to patients even though they could be a distortion of reality. For example, some patients interpret every ache or pain as a sign that the cancer is coming back: some patients believe strongly that no matter what happens the cancer is going to kill them, even in the absence of any active disease.

The key to changing this pattern of negative thinking is to try to help patients to identify the underlying thoughts that are contributing to their feelings. Having identified the negative thoughts, it is possible to examine what distortions there may be in their thinking. When thinking errors have been identified, the goal then lies in looking at how patients can challenge their negative and unrealistic thoughts and change them to something more positive. This raises a number of questions for the counsellor or therapist:

What kind of thinking errors or distortions do patients typically make?

How can counselling help to elucidate and bring to the surface these thoughts, which are contributing to the distress?

What communication process is necessary in order to encourage patients away from negative thoughts to a more positive and fighting view?

Moorey and Greer's excellent book (1989) clearly describes some of the classic thinking errors that people can make.

All or nothing thinking. The world is seen in very black and white terms, for example, 'If I can't be cured I might as well die now' or 'If I can't have my health back to what it was before the diagnosis, then I can't possibly enjoy life'.

Selective attention. Only those things that are negative are seen or heard, and it is not possible to see other aspects to the situation; for example, the anticipated unpleasant side effects of chemotherapy prevent the patient from seeing the possible long-term benefits.

Shoulds and oughts. A set of rules in one's head about what ought to be, for example, 'Even though I don't feel well, I should still be looking after my family' or 'I should be coping better than this, so I must be a useless person'.

Negative predictions. In this instance, although cancer carries with it a great deal of uncertainty, there is an assumption that the worst is going to happen, for example, 'I know the treatment won't work' or 'If I have a mastectomy my partner won't ever find me sexually attractive'.

Getting patients to change the way they think in order to help to reduce distress is often referred to as **cognitive restructuring**. This is the process of challenging irrational beliefs and replacing them with more realistic and adaptive ones; raising peoples' awareness of the existence of irrational beliefs, identifying these and then attempting to change or replace them. The process involves them in learning how to monitor their negative automatic thoughts – that is, they need to be able to identify beliefs that are irrational.

There are a number of steps to this cognitive therapy and the first is to introduce patients to the **skills model**, the idea that to learn coping strategies is similar to learning any new skill. It requires that they understand the steps involved in acquiring the skill, monitor their performance and then progress through feedback and to modify what they do accordingly. A useful analogy that can be used is learning to drive a car, as most people have some experience of this. This is not so banal as it may sound because it helps to explicate the skills model and thereby facilitates the process of monitoring negative automatic thoughts as a prerequisite for changing how one thinks. The aim is to introduce the patient to the cognitive model as a preliminary step to encouraging change. To achieve this it is helpful to emphasize that negative thoughts spring to mind without any effort, are easy to believe, are often not true, can be difficult to stop and are almost always unhelpful. People may find these negative thoughts difficult to spot to start with and the first step is to recognize them. They can be encouraged to keep track of them and examine how unrealistic or unhelpful they are. Examples can be given to illustrate the model. For instance, someone with cancer feels a twinge in the hip. They immediately think, 'I've got cancer in my bones'. This is a **negative automatic thought** as they have jumped to the worst possible conclusion, which is referred to as **catastrophizing**. Not surprisingly, they feel anxious. The thought, 'I've got cancer in my bones', can be challenged by the **rational response**, such as 'I had arthritis in my hip long before I got cancer. The last check-up showed the cancer hadn't spread. I'm misinterpreting ordinary aches and pains'. This can reduce the strength of the belief that the cancer has spread and the associated anxiety.

It is then possible to introduce the notion of **monitoring** these negative thoughts so that a clear picture can be obtained of the extent to which they contribute to levels of distress being experienced. By encouraging people to focus on the role such thoughts play in relation to their emotions they can begin the process of changing them. Giving people a homework exercise that requires them to 'catch the thoughts' can be very helpful at this point in the counselling process.

It is clear from the following example how most people thinking in this kind of way would end up feeling anxious and unhappy. Once people have understood the relationship between thoughts and emotions they can learn to replace negative thoughts with more helpful positive thoughts. At this point they can be encouraged to ask some questions when they begin to have thoughts that they suspect may be negative:

> Does the thought make them feel more anxious or depressed?
>
> Does it stop them from doing what they want to do? Is it true?
>
> Is there another way they can look at the situation?

They can learn to replace these thought with something more positive. For example:

Negative thought: 'I can feel a pain in my breast, the cancer is coming back'

Positive answer: 'Lumps that are cancerous are not usually painful and the scan showed everything was clear.'

Not everyone can make use of cognitive techniques such as those described here. Some proclaim an abhorrence of anything that sounds like 'positive thinking'. Others may not grasp the cognitive model; they may have little personal insight or they may feel so overwhelmed by their problems that they feel 'locked in' to their depression and anxiety. In such circumstances, behavioural techniques such as activity scheduling may bring some relief. However, for a minority of people neither nondirective counselling nor more structured cognitive methods is successful in relieving distress. Such patients may benefit from psychotropic medication as the first line of treatment.

There is some evidence that for more profoundly depressed patients a suitable model for treatment would be to offer antidepressants initially and then as symptoms begin to lift it may be possible to introduce psychological methods and effect a more long-lasting change in the patient's coping (Tarrier and Maguire 1984). Psychological techniques that involve the teaching of coping strategies can then provide patients with self-help skills that they can use should they experience future crises. The use of brief cognitive–behavioural therapy has been evaluated in a large randomized clinical trial and was found to be efficacious in reducing anxiety (Greer *et al.* 1992). More recent evidence indicates that it also has longer-term benefits (Moorey *et al.* 1994).

11
Group Therapy

The number of professionally led therapy groups has increased, and as a method of helping people with cancer this is a useful option to consider. The provision of psychological care in a support group is likely to be increasingly popular because many people with cancer prefer this kind of help and the group format can be cost-effective. Although there are an increasing number of self-help groups now available for people with cancer, this chapter will focus on professionally led groups.

What Type of Group?

There are a variety of therapeutic models, and no strong evidence that one approach is better than another; therapeutic model and method need to be tailored to specific needs. Support groups available to people with cancer tend to fall into two categories: the brief psychoeducational approach and the supportive psychotherapy group using nondirective techniques. They are not mutually exclusive because aspects of one approach can often be found in the other.

Psychoeducational groups

Psychoeducational groups are brief, problem-focused and didactic. A few controlled studies have been published that describe and evaluate these groups. Fawzy *et al.* (1990) describe a six-week structured intervention that includes teaching problem-solving skills, stress management, relaxation and health education, with accompanying handouts for participants. The groups run on a weekly basis for one and a half hours over a six-week period. Benefits include a reduction in depression and mood disturbance, with participants tending to use more active coping methods post-therapy. Cunningham's programme uses a standard psychoeducational format, teaching self-help techniques that can be delivered with equal effect as an intensive weekend or as a six-week group with weekly meetings (Cunningham *et al.* 1995).

The programme led by Stolbach and Lorman (1994) includes active behavioural problem-solving, relaxation, teaching about stress and stress management; it is usually delivered over an eight-week period in weekly two-hour sessions. Results indicate an improvement in coping and quality of life. Berglund *et al.* (1993) offer a programme of eleven two-hour sessions that includes physical and coping skills training along with information giving. Physical and psychological benefits are observed and participants increase their social activities. Kissane *et al.* (1997) use a structured model that draws on the cognitive–behavioural approach with notable effectiveness, demonstrating that an approach used successfully on an individual basis (Greer *et al.* 1992) can be adapted to a group format.

Nondirective groups

Nondirective groups tend to emphasize experiential aspects, with mutual support between participants a high priority. Spiegel's programme (Spiegel and Yalom 1978; Spiegel 1985) is an example. Women with advanced breast cancer discuss issues such as the demystification of dying, putting death into perspective, clarifying remaining life goals and coping with their own impending death. The efficacy of this model is well established in terms of benefits to mental health and quality of life. Effective application to other diagnostic groups at different stages of disease awaits further research. These groups tend to require a greater commitment of time for participants and facilitators as they often run weekly for some months. However, Phillips and Osborne (1989) describe an experientially based group with only six sessions. There the focus is on resolution of psychological issues and dissipation of negative feelings. Existential themes cover isolation, relationships, life/death challenges, choice and responsibility.

Other groups

The above gives a flavour of the differing approaches available rather than a complete overview. More complete reviews can be found in Cella and Yellen (1993), Fawzy *et al.* (1995), Harman (1991), Krupnick *et al.* (1993), Spiegel (1992) and Trijsburg *et al.* (1992). Vugia (1991) summarizes four main themes in support groups:

- intrapsychic themes: anger, fear of death, depression and worry
- interpersonal themes: marital/partner relationships, sexuality and the burden of disclosure
- social themes: isolation, stigma and lifestyle changes
- cancer-related themes: treatment side effects, treatment choices and doctor–patient relationships.

Running a Support Group

The approach described here for running a support group depends on the helper acting as a facilitator using structured cognitive–behavioural therapy (Watson *et al.* 1996). When planning a group support programme it is useful to consider at the outset how to audit this care in order to evaluate its benefits (see also Chapter 12). It is equally important to demonstrate that the intervention does no harm as to show that it does some good. Methods for the evaluation of group therapy are not dealt with here as the topic is beyond the scope of this book; however, the method of assessment chosen will depend on specific circumstances and needs. There is a substantial literature dealing with the methodology of assessment (including quality-of-life measures), and readers considering how to evaluate their groups might begin by using measures described in the outcome studies already cited. The organization of a support group can be divided into three parts: (1) planning and development, (2) implementation, and (3) review, revision and audit.

Planning a group

Helpers from any profession who are to facilitate a group will find it useful to arrange supervision with appropriate colleagues and to have this in place before any people with cancer are offered a place in the group. Practical matters to consider at the outset include:

- when and where the group is to meet and the ambience of the venue
- how people with cancer will be referred or recruited to the group
- whether the group will be closed (the same people attending) or open (anyone can attend when they choose)
- which diagnostic groups are to be targeted (disease-specific or any type of cancer)
- which disease stage will be the focus (early or advanced cancer)
- how information about the group will be communicated to the target population
- how and whether other professionals will be informed that patients are in the group
- what method of record-keeping needs to be set up
- what charges, if any, will be made and how these will be calculated and processed through the health care system
- whether the group conflicts with similar services in the host institution or locality

- preparation of materials (handouts, videos) for the programme

- training for those with limited experience of being a group
facilitator

- gathering information from other programmes and visits
to other establishments to learn how their programme
works

- setting up regular business meetings to promote programme development and ensure effective teamwork

- preparatory talks about the programme for teams and
professionals likely to refer patients

- method of pregroup assessment (motivation to attend and
engage, level of need)

- which people will lead or facilitate the group; a multi-
disciplinary approach is useful; a team might be made up
of nurses, occupational therapists, psychologists, social
workers, psychiatrists and others.

Some helpers will themselves have been treated for cancer
and their experience can be invaluable. However, careful selec-
tion and training of patient-helpers is important to ensure an
effective peer-counselling service is offered to people who will
be attending. While this list may seem daunting, it is very
worthwhile to complete some of this ground work before the
programme begins. Anyone who thinks they need not bother
with this preparatory work should seriously consider not
embarking on the work at all.

Implementation

Establishing 'housekeeping' for group participants is part of
implementation. This involves explaining the group rules and
giving information to people who choose to attend. This
includes:

- telling them when and where the group will meet

- time-keeping and the need to let the group facilitators know if someone is unable to attend

- what structure, if any, the group will have and what topics are likely to be covered

- letting people know they will all have an equal chance to speak in the group sessions but they will not be pressured to speak

- what is discussed in the group remains confidential so that people attending can feel free to express feelings and talk about things which are private

- whether the group is open (new members can join at any point) or closed (no new members will be allowed to join over the course of the group)

- for whom the group is intended, if this is not explicit in the advertising material or through the referral system

- clarifying whether partners or other carers can attend

- whether the group is time-limited (to a number of sessions) or ongoing

- what to expect (whether there are educational elements, whether the group activity is limited in any way and what will be required of them as participants)

- whether information about their attendance will be communicated to other professionals, what this information might be and what their rights are regarding this process.

Establishing the 'housekeeping' is part of the initial therapeutic contract and can usually be done at the first meeting.

Group cognitive–behavioural therapy

Cognitive–behavioural therapy has increased in popularity and given the accumulating evidence of its efficacy, is well worth considering. Training in cognitive–behavioural therapy is needed, but for those who wish to pursue this method, it is a worthwhile training commitment to make. However, not all group facilitators need to have a recognized qualification in this method. There will often be some passing on of skills by training members of the team, which will allow untrained staff to develop these skills with the passage of time.

The programme can be divided into four components: (a) ventilation of emotions; (b) coping skills such as activity scheduling, challenging negative automatic thoughts, distraction, stress management and relaxation; (c) information-giving; and (d) facilitating the development of mutual support.

(a) **Ventilation of emotions.** As described in individual therapy (Chapter 10), the ventilation of problems and emotions is an important feature of the support group and is encouraged early in the programme. Failure to allow adequate emotional ventilation at an early stage may inhibit the development of a collaborative relationship between facilitator and group members and can stymie the introduction of more structured and didactic therapeutic activities. The sharing of emotions among group members can be arduous and demanding of them and needs careful facilitation. Any specific individual problems, concerns and feelings are brought into the group forum in such a way that there is shared discussion. Failure to do this can make the group format feel rather like individual therapy taking place within a group, and the benefit of the group dynamic is lost.

Ventilation within the group format involves the facilitator in imposing some order on the communication process. Methods of achieving this include:

Paraphrasing: 'So you seem to be saying that you feel...'

Normalizing: 'Others in the group seem to be saying that they have felt like this...'

Time-limit warnings: 'We're about to run out of time on this topic but we'll come back to it...'

Sharing the load: 'These are strong emotions; how do others feel?'

Acceptance: 'Do you think it makes a difference that you don't all feel the same about this?'

Acknowledging the burden of sharing: 'Sometimes it can be very hard to listen to others talking about their feelings. How do you feel about this?'

Responsibility: 'We may all feel the pressure to help others with their problems, but do you think it's necessary to come up with solutions to them?'

Insight: 'Do you recognize these feelings in yourself?'

Summarizing: 'Let's just review what we've discussed...'.

No matter how thoughtful the helper's facilitation of the process of ventilation, there will always be some participants whose problems might be better addressed in individual therapy, and there will always be people whose typical coping response (Chapter 3) will cause them to feel uncomfortable with these discussions. Additional individual sessions may be indicated for some people.

(b) **Coping skills**. Cognitive–behavioural therapy is a pragmatic problem-solving treatment. Early in the group programme participants can be introduced to the idea of developing new coping skills, planning for change and reviewing progress. This usually involves goal-setting, prioritizing and recording progress using formal (record sheet) or informal (review discussion) methods. Discussion of obstacles and barriers to plans, goals and methods should be included. Brainstorming discussions might revolve around methods for dealing with barriers to coping and thinking creatively. Group members are often pleased to have an opportunity to share their experiences while learning new coping skills. Often they can talk about differences in the way they have approached a problem, and this can engender a feeling of mutual support.

These discussions can be facilitated through comments like:

So Sally, you've already had this problem but you tackled it some time ago. How did that work out and what did you do?

What we understand is that Sally and Mary have both had this problem but others haven't. Is that right?

The basic techniques of cognitive–behavioural therapy are described in Chapter 10 and can easily be implemented in the group: activity scheduling, monitoring and challenging negative automatic thoughts, distraction and cognitive restructuring. The main difference between implementation in individual sessions and in group therapy is the sharing of thoughts and feelings by group members and the mutual support that comes from tackling problems together.

Where participants feel inhibited or awkward about discussing their own problems, it can be useful to use anonymous case examples. Presenting details of an anonymous case and opening the discussion by saying, 'What do you think this woman's negative automatic thoughts are?', will often lead naturally into disclosure of others' thoughts and how they compare. The therapeutic power of the group lies in the credibility members have with each other. Discussion of how to move forward in dealing with problems is greatly facilitated by the feeling of 'I've been there, I know what it's like'.

Mrs. D talked in the group about the lack of disclosure of her diagnosis to others and that she wanted to keep it private. She felt this faced her with a quandary and wondered if it was the right thing to do. This generated a discussion in the group about the costs and benefits of telling others you have cancer, some of which she had been unable to see or experience. She was able to share some of their experiences and ask how it was for others. She was also faced with a group of other people in the same situation who challenged her reasons for doing this as well as supporting her in her fears and apprehensions. 'I know, I felt like that, but...' Through this discussion she was able to consider her decision, look at the emotions driving it and eventually deal with them and escape from her quandary.

(c) **Information-giving**. Many structured groups that are didactic in nature involve the giving of information about aspects of medical and nursing care. This may range from passing on information about the disease and the treatment programmes to the provision of practical advice such as the location of rehabilitation services and information booklets. The group forum should preferably not be used to discuss specific medical problems that are better dealt with by the medical team. How to assess this medical information and any communication problems between patient and doctor, however, are legitimately on the group agenda. Teaching communication skills to people with cancer may be at least as important as teaching doctors these skills, thereby acknowledging that doctor–patient communication can be improved if patients feel empowered to communicate more effectively. In this way they may feel better able to get the information they want about their disease or treatment.

(d) **Mutual support**. What distinguishes the group from other forms of helping is the ability of people with cancer to gain access to a system of sharing. From the unburdening of emotions with others in a similar situation to the swapping of ideas about how to resolve problems, the 'all in the same boat' ethos builds group cohesion. Although at times the facilitator will draw attention to individual differences, when the shared issues are emphasized the group begins to gel and, as one patient put it,

> *When we're away from the group we all have different lifestyles, but when we're here we know we all have cancer and can say things to each other that we might not say to others, including our families.*

The social element should not be forgotten. Friendships are struck up and communication goes on between group members outside the group. Group members sometimes become co-therapists, helping others outside the formal structure of the group. The facilitator's role is to recognize this process and support it when support is needed.

Review and audit

A businesslike approach to running a support group involves implementing review and audit, and this works at two levels. One is the formal evaluation of benefits of patient participation in terms of changes in emotions and ways of tackling problems. This can be done by using outcome measures that assess aspects of psychopathology, coping and quality of life. Records of who has participated and when can be reviewed in order to clarify whether the programme is cost-effective and attendance is being maintained at a workable level. At a second level, sessions can be reviewed by the facilitators either with each other or with a colleague:

- how were problematic communications dealt with in the discussions?
- whether a specific intervention by a facilitator was or was not needed
- were there difficulties in getting discussions going and why did this occur?
- was animosity or discord evident?
- did the facilitator's intervention defuse difficult incidents?
- did the discussions become poorly balanced by one or two participants dominating?
- were techniques effective in controlling the flow of discussion?

These review sessions are best done soon after a group session while discussions are still fresh; they are important not only because they may improve the facilitation of future groups but also because facilitators occasionally need help themselves with their efforts. The work of running a support group will be an enjoyable experience for most facilitators if they too feel there is a system to support them.

12
Professional Issues

Setting up a Service

People who find themselves counselling cancer patients may be working from a range of organizations, including voluntary groups, social services, general practice, hospitals and community agencies (not a comprehensive list). Despite this variability in work base, there are some general principles to guide the development of a new service or to act as the basis for considering revision to an established service that is to be extended to include those with cancer.

It is helpful to work as closely as possible with the institutions where patients receive their medical care. The reason for this is obvious but still worth stating. It is far better when counselling cancer patients to be well informed of their medical progress and treatment, and to get this information from the doctors organizing their care. For example, discussions with patients about how they cope with their disease and treatment, and especially how they cope with their prognosis, can be done more effectively if you know what is going on. Whether the patient is responding by denying the seriousness of the disease is difficult to judge if you have only the patient's report to act upon.

Having said that, it may be possible to provide a useful service away from the source of the medical treatment but liaising closely with patients' general practitioners. It is not possible to offer a fully effective service if there is no communication with those who have charge of patients' medical treatment; although voluntary organizations have something to contribute to the psychological care of the cancer patient, counselling services are best offered from within the National Health Service. The fact that they have not been widely available has meant that other agencies have stepped in to bridge the gap. In an increasingly expensive health service, it is hard to find financial support for this dimension of patient care despite the fact that it is often recognized as valuable. For a disease like cancer where treatment is frequently offered to prolong life and to assuage symptoms rather than to cure, there is a desperate need to recognize the importance of the psychological dimension of care and not simply to see it as a 'soft option'.

The first step, therefore, in setting up a service is to convince potential referrers that psychological support and counselling are worth providing. In the present climate, this often means finding ways of 'selling' the service. This may mean convincing referrers not only that patients' quality of life may be improved but also that there are financial benefits. For example, will psychological or counselling services help to reduce patients' length of stay in hospital? Will it reduce the number of unnecessary visits to doctors? Will it reduce the number of drugs required, or the need for referral to social services? A good psychological service can potentially do all of these. For example, a study by Robson *et al.* (1984) indicated that psychological services in primary care lead to reductions in patients' general practitioner consultation rates and the number of drugs prescribed. There is evidence that investment in psychological and counselling services has long-term financial benefits (Schlesinger *et al.* 1983) in addition to the more obvious benefits of improved quality of life.

Service Evaluation

The potential benefits, discussed above, are not always obvious, nor should it be assumed that we do not need to demonstrate the efficacy of what we do to reduce psychological problems and distress. It is important to maintain audit and evaluation of services in order to provide evidence of benefits. Audit also serves to correct unworkable aspects of a service. Therefore, an important step in the setting up of a service is to build in a system of evaluation of outcome (Goodare 1994).

At the Royal Marsden NHS Trust, a randomized controlled trial was conducted (Greer *et al.* 1992) to compare the cognitive–behavioural method (described in Chapter 10) with routine care. This comparison showed an advantage over routine care in terms of reduction of anxiety up to one year post-treatment. Randomized controlled trials are, however, quite complex, requiring a strict research procedure. Sometimes financial or ethical constraints prevent this type of strict evaluation. Where it is not possible to conduct a controlled trial, it is necessary to find other methods of evaluation, including single case designs. Methods of evaluating service should include a range of measures such as:

- psychological morbidity, especially depression and anxiety
- the cost of the service
- its social benefits in terms of social and occupational functioning
- the number of visits and the structure of the service provided
- quality-of-life evaluation.

Measures of Psychological Morbidity

Current measures in use are those that focus on the evaluation of depression and anxiety. For populations of medical patients, questions should preferably exclude somatic symptoms as these may be caused by the mental state, disease progress or treament side effects. For example, loss of appetite is symptomatic of depression but also occurs when patients are receiving chemotherapy. Where the disease or treatment are stable, however, other more widely used measures should not be excluded. Short questionnaire assessments are available that are well validated, such as the Hospital Anxiety and Depression Scale (HADS) (Zigmond and Snaith 1983), the General Health Questionnaire (GHQ) (Goldberg and Williams 1988) and the Profile of Mood States (POMS) (McNair *et al.* 1971), but the best method by far is a full mental state examination aimed at a formal psychiatric diagnosis. There is no inherent mystique to conducting a mental state examination and it is possible for a wide range of staff to learn to do this with a minimum of training (Maguire *et al.* 1980). All staff who will be regularly involved in the psychological care of people with cancer should be encouraged to obtain full training in making a mental state examination using a clinical interview and should not have to rely solely on self-report questionnaires.

Economic Measures

It is important, especially in a state-run health service or a programme of managed care, to include in any audit the running costs. This issue will not be new to those who work within the formal health services. However, there are other areas of economic evaluation worth considering that do not perhaps readily spring to mind. For instance, it is worth looking at:

- the extent to which the service can reduce demand on inpatient beds
- the extent to which drug bills can be minimized by a psychological rather than a psychiatric intervention
- the extent to which we can reduce the need for patients to spend time away from their work.

Supervision

Supervision needs are determined by a number of factors including helpers' feelings of comfort with psychological techniques and their level of experience in working with people who have cancer. Even the most experienced counsellors welcome the regular opportunity to discuss difficult or complex cases. Supervision is most often available from colleagues or, in some instances, arrangements can be made for two people to provide mutual peer supervision. Sometimes counselling supervision groups can be formed. These are particularly helpful where counsellors work in isolation. Counsellors from other hospitals or specialist centres may wish to meet in a group with those from different organizations or departments. Such groups can operate on a peer-counselling basis or can be coordinated by a facilitator or group leader.

Whenever supervision occurs, the contract should be clearly specified, including the length and frequency of meetings. It is also important for supervisors to clarify the limits of their expertise. Supervision is an ongoing relationship giving the supervisee the opportunity to discuss cases as they unfold over time. Supervision is an integral element of counselling and should always be available. No counsellor should attempt to set up a service without first ensuring provision for supervision.

There is also the issue of the counsellor's own psychological needs. Involvement in other peoples' emotional life can be taxing and demanding. Although it is important to maintain optimal objectivity, it is not always possible to remain immune to the issues. Helpers who find themselves becoming very affected by their patients' problems should themselves seek advice and support. On occasion, counsellors do cry with their patients and there are differing opinions on whether this is desirable. In general, it does not help to become over-involved emotionally in patients' problems. There are too many patients requiring support and to help them we need to be able to stand sufficiently outside events to maintain objectivity. Counsellors or helpers who cannot do this risk burnout. Such issues can be discussed with a supervisor should the problem arise.

Confidentiality

The issue of confidentiality is a matter of professional responsibility. Patients need to be able to disclose fully and in confidence, and this is a central element in any trusting relationship. Patients may entrust their counsellor with intimate details of their personal life, disclosing things that they expect to go no further. This may be implicit on occasions to some people entering counselling, but if there is any doubt, it may be important to specify clearly that information they impart to you will be treated in confidence and, if not, what the limitations of confidentiality might be. For the purposes of supervision, patients' identities should be protected or anonymized in order to ensure the contract of confidentiality is not broken. There are a few exceptions: if the patient gives permission to break confidentiality, if the helper wishes or needs to refer on the patient to another counsellor or mental health professional and this has been agreed, or if either the patient or someone else will be put at risk if information is not passed on.

All mental health professionals are called upon to communicate about their patients' mental health to other professionals caring for them, and this is usually done in order to ensure that patients receive the appropriate level of care. However, it is possible to communicate effectively with other professionals about patients' progress without necessarily undermining confidentiality. It is important for patients to understand the basis of their relationship with a counsellor in terms of maintaining confidentiality, but it is equally important that they should not assume that confidentiality is an absolute. Where the patient has been referred to a counsellor for an opinion on their mental health, then there is a responsibility to provide that opinion to the referrer, providing the patient is willing to be seen. If there is any uncertainty about this, it can be clarified to patients that the aim of providing feedback to referrers is in order to provide better care for them, as their mental health needs impact upon other areas of their care.

The Counselling Contract

Once an evaluation of needs and mental state has been made, it is then possible to formulate a treatment plan and to describe to the patient what is on offer. This process of establishing the contract usually involves giving details of the timing and frequency of sessions along with the usual length of each session. The aims of counselling should be specified where possible, and the counsellor may make the issue of confidentiality clear at this point. The contract with patients is verbal and not written, although it can be written if this seems appropriate. However, it should not be seen as inflexible and it should be possible to renegotiate the basis for the relationship if things change.

Most counsellors keep notes to help them to maintain continuity and in order to remember important details from session to session, including notes on the psychological treatment plan, should there be one. Some counsellors consider it appropriate to declare that such notes are being kept; others do not. If the notes are used solely for the counsellor's use and are to enable the counselling process, then it may not be necessary to declare this explicitly. However, if there is any doubt, it may be simpler when seeing patients to say that you are going to make some notes but these are for your own use in order for you to recall important points in the sessions.

The contract provides a framework for counselling and is not only helpful to the patient but can also help the carer in formulating the psychological treatment plan. Where possible, it should be expressed in an informal and supportive manner and should facilitate the establishment of a trusting relationship with the patient.

References

Abt, V., McGurran, M.C. and Heintz, L. (1978) The impact of mastectomy on sexual self-image, attitudes and behavior. *J. Sex Educ. Ther.* **4**, 43–46.

Altmaier, E.M., Ross, W.E. and Moore, K. (1982) A pilot investigation of the psychological function of patients with anticipatory vomiting. *Cancer* **49**, 201–204.

Andrykowski, M.A., Jacobsen, P.B., Marks, E., Garfinkle, K., Hakes, T.B., Kaufman, R.J., Currie, V.E., Holland, J.C. and Redd, W.H. (1988) Prevalence, predictors and course of anticipatory nausea in women receiving adjuvant chemotherapy for breast cancer. *Cancer* **62**, 2607–2613.

Asher, R. (1972) *Talking Sense.* Tunbridge Wells: Pitman.

Atkinson, J.M. (1993) The patient as sufferer. *Br. J. Med. Psych.* **66**, 113–140.

Auchincloss, S.S. (1989) Sexual dysfunction in cancer patients: issues in evaluation and treatment. In: J.C. Holland and J.H. Rowland (eds), *Handbook of psycho-oncology.* Oxford: Oxford University Press, pp. 383–413.

Auden, W.H. (1976) 'Miss Gee'. *Collected Poems.* London: Faber & Faber.

BACUP (1994a) *Understanding radiotherapy.* London: BACUP.

BACUP (1994b) *Understanding chemotherapy.* London: BACUP.

BACUP (1994c) *Coping with hair loss.* London: BACUP.

Baider, L., Cooper, C.L. and De-Nour, A.K. (eds) (1996) *Cancer and the family.* Chichester: Wiley.

Baider, L., Peretz, T. and De-Nour, A.K. (1997) The effect of behavioral intervention on the psychological distress of Holocaust survivors with cancer. *Psychother. Psychosom.* **66**, 44–49.

Bard, M. and Sutherland, A.M. (1955) Psychological impact of cancer and its treatment IV. Adaptation to radical mastectomy. *Cancer* **8**, 656–672.

Beck, A.T. (1976) *Cognitive therapy and the emotional disorders.* New York: International Universities Press.

Bellet, P.S. and Maloney, M.J. (1991) The importance of empathy as an interviewing skill in medicine. *J. Am. Med. Assoc.* **266**, 1831–1832.

Bennett, M. and Alison, D. (1996) Discussing the diagnosis and prognosis with cancer patients. *Postgrad. Med. J.* **72**, 25–29.

Benson, J. and Britten, N. (1996) Respecting the autonomy of cancer patients when talking with their families: qualitative analysis of semistructured interviews with patients. *Br. Med. J.* **313**, 729–731.

Berglund, G.C. *et al.* (1993) Starting again: a comparison study of a group rehabilitation program for cancer patients. *Acta Oncol.* **32**, 15–21.

Berne, E. (1972) *What do you say after you say hello? The psychology of human destiny.* New York: Grove Press.

Bernstein, W.C. (1972) Sexual dysfunction following radical surgery for cancer of rectum and sigmoid colon. *Med. Asp. Hum. Sexuality* March 6, 156–163.

Bird, B. (1973). *Talking with patients*, 2nd edn. Philadelphia: J.B. Lippincott.

Bloom, J.R. (1982) Social support accommodation to stress and adaptation to breast cancer. *Soc.Sci. Med.* **16**, 1329–1330.

Bluglass, K. (1991) Care of the cancer patient's family. In: M. Watson (ed.), *Cancer patient care: psychosocial treatment methods*. Cambridge: BPS Books and Cambridge University Press, pp. 159–189.

Boehnert, C.E. (1986) Surgical outcome in 'death-minded' patients. *Psychosomatics* **27**, 638–642.

Bourke, R. (1984) Thriving with a stoma. *Nurs. Mirror* **159**, v-vi.

Branch, W.T. and Malik, T.K. (1993) Using 'windows of opportunity' in brief interviews to understand patients' concerns. *J. Am. Med. Assoc.* **269**, 1667–1668.

Brewin, T.B. (1977) The cancer patient: communication and morale. *Br. Med. J.* ii, 1623–1627.

Brewin, T.B. (1991) Three ways of giving bad news. *Lancet* **337**, 1207–1209.

Brewin, T.B. and Sparshott, M. (1996) *Relating to the relatives: breaking bad news, communication and support.* Oxford: Radcliffe Medical Press.

Buckman, R. (1984). Breaking bad news: why is it still so difficult? *Br. Med. J.* **288**, 1597–1599.

Buckman, R. (1986) Communicating with the patient. In: B.A. Stoll and A.D. Weisman (eds), *Coping with cancer stress*. Dordrecht: Martinus Nijhoff, pp. 165–173.

Buckman, R. (1989) Communicating with cancer patients. *Practitioner* **233**, 1393–1394.

Buckman, R. (1994) *Lost for words: how to talk to someone with cancer*. London: BACUP.

Buckman, R. (1996) Talking to patients about cancer: no excuse now for not doing it. *Br. Med. J.* **313**, 699–700.

Buckman, R. and Kason, Y. (1993) *How to break bad news – a practical guide for healthcare professionals*. London: Macmillan.

Bunston, T., Elliott, M. and Rapuch, S. (1993) A psychosocial summary flow sheet: facilitating the coordination of care, enhancing the quality of care. *J. Palliative Care* **9**, 14–22.

Burton, M.V. and Parker, R.W. (1994) Satisfaction of breast cancer patients with their medical and psychological care. *J. Psychosoc. Oncol.* **12**, 41–63.

Burton, M.V. and Parker, R.W. (1995) A randomized controlled trial of preoperative psychological preparation for mastectomy. *Psycho-oncology* **4**, 1–19.

Burton, M.V. and Parker, R.W. (1997) Psychological aspects of cancer surgery: surgeons' attitudes and opinions. *Psycho-oncology* **6**, 47–64.

Butow, P.N., Dunn, S.M., Tattersall, M.H. and Jones, Q.J. (1994) Patient participation in the cancer consultation: evaluation of a question prompt sheet. *Ann. Oncol.* **5**, 199–204.

Butow, P.N., Kazemi, J.H., Beeney, L.J., Griffin, A.M., Dunn, S.M. and Tattersall, M.H.N. (1996) When the diagnosis is cancer: patient communication experiences and preferences. *Cancer* **77**, 2630–2637.

Cancer Research Campaign (1989). *Mortality. Factsheet 3.1*. London: Cancer Research Campaign.

Casement, P. (1985) *On learning from the patient*. London: Tavistock/Routledge.

Cassell, E. (1976). *The healer's art*. Philadelphia: J.B. Lippincott.

Cassell, E. (1985) *Talking with patients*, Volume 2. Cambridge: MIT Press.

Cassidy, S. (1986) Emotional distress in terminal cancer: discussion paper. *J. R. Soc. Med.* **79**, 717–720.

Cassidy, S. (1991) Terminal care. In: M. Watson (ed.), *Cancer patient care: psychosocial treatment methods*. Cambridge: BPS Books and Cambridge University Press, pp. 136–158.

Cella, D. and Yellen, S. (1993) Cancer support groups: The state of the art. *Cancer Pract.* **1**, 56–61.

Centeno-Cortes, C. and Nunez-Olarte, J.M. (1994) Questioning diagnosis disclosure in terminal cancer patients: a prospective study evaluating patients' responses. *Palliative Med.* **8**, 39–44.

Channel 4 Television (1994) *An interview with Dennis Potter.* An edited transcript of Melvyn Bragg's interview with Dennis Potter, broadcast on the 5th of April 1994. Potter died on 7 June 1994.

Charles-Edwards, A. (1983) *The nursing care of the dying patient: in the midst of life.* Beaconsfield: Beaconsfield Publishers.

Clark, G.T., Cole, G. and Enzle, S. (1990) Complicated grief reactions in women who were sexually abused in childhood. *J. Psychosoc. Oncol.* **8**, 87–97.

Classen, C., Koopman, C., Angell, K. and Spiegel, D. (1996) Coping styles associated with psychological adjustment to advanced breast cancer. *Health Psychol.* **15**, 434–437.

Corradi, R.B. (1983) Psychological regression with illness. *Psychosomatics* **24**, 353–362.

Cramond, W.A. (1970) Psychotherapy of the dying patient. *Br. Med. J.* **3**, 389–393.

Creagan, E.T. (1994) How to break bad news – and not devastate the patient. *Mayo Clin. Proc.* **69**, 1015–1017.

Creagan, E.T. (1997) Attitude and disposition: do they make a difference in cancer survival? *Mayo Clin. Proc.* **72**, 160–164.

Crisp, A. (1986) Undergraduate training for communication in medical practice. *J. R. Soc. Med.* **79**, 568–574.

Crits-Christoph, P. and Barber, J.P. (eds) (1991) *Handbook of short-term dynamic psychotherapy.* New York: Basic Books.

Cull, A. (1990) Invited review: psychological aspects of cancer and chemotherapy. *J. Psychosom. Res.* **34**, 129–140.

Cunningham, A.J., Edmonds, C.V., Jenkins, G. and Lockwood, G. (1995) A randomized comparison of two forms of a brief, group psycho-educational program for cancer patients: weekly sessions vs. a weekend intensive. *Int. J. Psychiatr. Med.* **25**, 173–189.

Dean, C. (1987) Psychiatric morbidity following mastectomy: preoperative predictors and types of illness. *J. Psychosom. Res.* **31**, 385–392.

Department of Health Expert Advisory Group on Cancer to the Chief Medical Officer of England and Wales (1995) *A policy framework for commissioning cancer services* ['The Calman Report']. London: HMSO.

Derogatis, L.R., Morrow, G.R., Fetting, J., Penman, D., Piasetsky, S., Schmale, A.M., Henrichs, M. and Carnicke, C.L.M. (1983) The prevalence of psychiatric disorders among cancer patients. *J. Am. Med. Assoc.* **249**, 751–757.

Dlin, B.M. (1973) Emotional aspects of colostomy and ileostomy. In:

A.E. Lindner (ed.), *Emotional factors in gastrointestinal illness.* New York: Elsevier. pp. 113–134.

Dosanjh, N., Marshall, H. and Yazdani, A. (1977) Mental health needs of young Asian women in Newham. Paper presented at the *Annual Conference of the BPS Primary Care Special Interest Group,* York, 6 June.

Dubovsky, S.L. and Weissberg, M.P. (1982) *Clinical psychiatry in primary care,* 2nd edn. Baltimore: Williams & Wilkins.

Eardley, A. (1985) Patients and radiotherapy. 1. Expectations of treatment. 2. Patients' experiences of treatment. 3. Patients' experiences after discharge. 4. How can patients be helped? *Radiography* 51, 324–326; 52, 17–22.

Engel, G.L. (1968) A life setting conducive to illness: The giving up–given up complex. *Ann. Int. Med.* 69, 293–300.

Engel, G.L. (1977) The need for a new medical model: a challenge for biomedicine. *Science* 196, 129–136.

Espinosa, E., Gonzalez, B.M., Zamora, P., Ordonez, A. and Arranz, P. (1996) Doctors also suffer when giving bad news to cancer patients. *Support Care Cancer* 4, 61–63.

Euster, S. (1984) Adjusting to an adult family member's cancer. In: H.B. Roback (ed.), *Helping patients and their families cope with medical problems: a guide to therapeutic group work in clinical settings.* San Francisco: Jossey-Bass, pp. 428–452.

Everson, S.A., Goldberg, D.E. and Kaplan, G.A. (1996) Hopelessness and risk of mortality and incidence of myocardial infarction and cancer. *Psychosom. Med.* 58, 113–121.

Fallowfield, L.J. and Clark, A.W. (1994) Delivering bad news in gastroenterology. *Am. J. Gastroenterol.* 89, 473–479.

Fallowfield, L.J., Ford, S. and Lewis, S. (1995) No news is not good news: information preferences of patients with cancer. *Psycho-oncology* 4, 197–202.

Faulkner, A. and Maguire, P. (1996) *Talking to cancer patients and their relatives.* Oxford: Oxford University Press.

Fawzy, F., Cousins, N., Fawzy, N.W., Kemeny, M.E., Elashoff, R. and Morton, D. (1990) A structured psychiatric intervention for cancer patients: Changes over time in methods of coping and affective disturbance. *Arch. Gen. Psychiatr.* 47, 720–725.

Fawzy, F., Fawzy, N.W., Arndt, L.A. and Pasnau, R.O. (1995) Critical review of psychosocial interventions in cancer care. *Arch. Gen. Psychiatry* 52, 100–113.

Fisher, S.G. (1983) The psychosexual effects of cancer and cancer treatment. *Oncol. Nurs. Forum* 10, 63–68.

Fletcher, C.M. (1973) Communication with patients. In: *Communication in Medicine.* London: Nuffield Provincial Hospitals Trust, pp. 7–32.

Fletcher, C. (1980) Listening and talking to patients II: the clinical interview. *Br. Med. J.* **281**, 931–933.

Ford, S., Fallowfield, L., Hall, A. and Lewis, S. (1995) The influence of audiotapes on patient participation in the cancer consultation. *Eur. J. Cancer* **31A**, 2264–2269.

Freedman, B. (1993) Offering truth: one ethical approach to the uninformed cancer patient. *Arch. Int. Med.* **153**, 572–576.

Garfield, C.A. (1976) Foundations of psychosocial oncology: the terminal phase. *Front. Rad. Ther. Oncol.* **11**, 180–212.

Gates, C.C. (1988) The 'most significant other' in the care of the breast cancer patient. *CA: A Cancer J. for Clinicians* 38, 146–153.

Gendlin, E. (1962) *Experiencing and the creation of meaning.* New York: Free Press of Glencoe.

Gendlin, E. (1967) Therapeutic procedures with schizophrenics. In C.R. Rogers (ed.) *Thetherapeutic relationship and its impact: a study of psychotherapy with schizophrenics.* Madison, WN: University of Wisconsin Press.

Ger, L.P., Ho, S.T., Chiang, H.H. and Chen, W.W. (1996) Cancer patients' knowledge of their diagnoses. *J. Formos. Med. Assoc.* **95**, 605–611.

Geringer, E.S. and Stern, T.A. (1986) Coping with medical illness: The impact of personality types. *Psychosomatics* 27, 251–261.

Gilbar, O., Steiner, M. and Atad, J. (1995) Adjustment of married couples and unmarried women to gynaecological cancer. *Psycho-oncology* **4**, 203–211.

Gillis, L. (1972) *Human behaviour in illness,* 2nd edn. London: Faber.

Given, C.W., Stommel, M., Given, B., Osuch, J., Kurtz, M. and Kurtz, J.C. (1993) The influence of cancer patient symptoms, functional states on patient depression and family caregiver reaction and depression. *Health Psychol.* 12, 277–285.

Gloeckner, M.R. (1983) Partner reaction following ostomy surgery. *J. Sex Marital Ther.* 9, 182–190.

Goddard, R. (1991) *Take no farewell.* Corgi Books.

Goldberg, D. and Williams, P. (1988) *A user's guide to the general health questionnaire.* London: NFER-Nelson.

Goldberg, R.J. (1984) Disclosure of information to adult cancer patients: issues and update. *J. Clin. Oncol.* 2, 948–955.

Goldberg, R.J. and Tull, R.M. (1983) *The psychosocial dimensions of cancer.* New York: Free Press.

Goldie, L. (1982) The ethics of telling the patient. *J. Med. Ethics* **8**, 128–133.

Goodare, H. (1994) Counseling people with cancer: questions and possibilities. *Advances* **10**, 4–17.

Gordon, T. (1970) *Parent effectiveness training.* New York: Wyden.

Gorlin, R. and Zucker, H.D. (1983) Physicians' reactions to patients: a key to teaching humanistic medicine. *New Eng. J. Med.* **308**, 1059–1063.

Gotay, C.C. (1996) Cultural variation in family adjustment to cancer. In: L. Baider, C.L. Cooper and A.K. De-Nour (eds), *Cancer and the family.* Chichester: Wiley, pp. 31–52.

Grassi, L. and Rosti, G. (1996) Psychiatric and psychosocial concomitants of abnormal illness behaviour in patients with cancer. *Psychother. Psychosom.* **65**, 246–252.

Greer, S. (1991) Stress and psychological aspects of cancers. In: *Reducing the risk of cancers. study pack.* Milton Keynes: The Open University.

Greer, S. (1992) The management of denial in cancer patients. *Oncology* **6**, 39–40.

Greer, S., Morris, T. and Pettingale, K.W. (1979) Psychological responses to breast cancer: effect on outcome. *Lancet* **ii**, 785–787.

Greer, S., Moorey, S., Baruch, J.D.R., Watson, M., Robertson, B., Mason, A., Rowden, L., Law, M. and Bliss, J. (1992) Adjuvant psychological therapy for patients with cancer: a prospective randomized trial. *Br. Med. J.* **304**, 675–680.

Grossman, S.A., Piantoadosi, S. and Covahey, C. (1994) Are informed consent forms that describe clinical oncology research protocols readable by most patients and their families? *J. Clin. Oncol.* **12**, 2211–2215.

Groves, J.E. (ed.) (1996) *Essential papers on short-term dynamic therapy.* New York: New York University Press.

Hainsworth, M.A., Eakes, G.G. and Burke, M.L. (1994) Coping with chronic sorrow. *Issues Ment. Health Nurs.* **15**, 59–66.

Halldorsdottir, S. and Hamrin, E. (1996) Experiencing existential changes: the lived experience of having cancer. *Cancer Nurs.* **19**, 29–36.

Harman, M. (1991) The use of group psychotherapy with cancer patients: A review of recent literature. *J. Specialists in Group Work,* **16**, 56–61.

Harrison, J., Haddad, P. and Maguire, P. (1995) The impact of cancer on key relatives: a comparison of relative and patient concerns. *Eur. J. Cancer* **31A**, 1736–1740.

Heim, E. (1991) Coping and adaptation in cancer. In: C. Cooper and M. Watson (eds), *Cancer and stress: Psychological, biological and coping studies.* Chichester: John Wiley, pp. 197–235.

Hermann, J.F. (1985) Psychosocial support: interventions for the physician. *Semin. Oncol.* **12**, 466–471.

Highfield, M.F. and Cason, C. (1983) Spiritual needs of patients: are they recognised? *Cancer Nurs.* **6**, 187–192.

Himmelhoch, J.M., Davies, R.K., Tucker, G.J. and Alderman, D. (1970) Butting heads: patients who refuse necessary procedures. *Psychiatr. Med.* **1**, 241–249.

Hogbin, B. and Fallowfield, L. (1989) Getting it taped: the ''bad news' consultation with cancer patients. *Br. J. Hosp. Med.* **41**, 330–333.

Holland, J. (1989). Radiotherapy. In: J.C. Holland and J.H. Rowland (eds), *Handbook of Psycho-oncology.* New York: Oxford University Press, pp. 134–145.

Holland, J.C. and Jacobs, E. (1986) Psychiatric sequelae following surgical treatment of breast cancer. *Adv. Psychosom. Med.* **15**, 109–123.

Holland, J.C. and Rowland, J.H. (1989) *Handbook of Psycho-oncology.* New York: Oxford University Press.

Hoy, A.M. (1985) Breaking bad news to patients. *Br. J. Hosp. Med.* **34**, 96–99.

Hughes, J. (1982) Emotional reactions to the diagnosis of and treatment of early breast cancer. *J. Psychosom. Res.* **26**, 277–283.

Hurny, C. and Holland, J. (1985) Psychosocial sequelae of ostomies in cancer patients. *CA: A Cancer J. for Clinicians* **35**, 170–183.

Jenkins, R.A. and Pargament, K.l. (1995) Religion and spirituality as resources for coping with cancer. *J. Psychosoc. Oncol.* **13**, 51–74.

Jewson, N.D. (1976) The disappearance of the sick-man from medical cosmology 1870–1970. *Sociology* **10**, 225–244.

Josephs, L. (1996) Women and trauma: a contemporary psychodynamic approach to traumatization for patients in the OB/GYN psychological consultation clinic. *Bull. Menn. Clinic* **60**, 22–38.

Kaplan, H.S. (1992) A neglected issue: the sexual side effects of current treatments for breast cancer. *J. Sex Marital Ther.* **18**, 3–19.

Kelly, P.T. (1987) Risk counselling for relatives of cancer patients: new information, new approaches. *J. Psychosocial Oncol.* **5**, 65–79.

Kissane, D.W., Bloch, S., Burns, W.l., Patrick, J.D., Wallace, C.S. and McKenzie, D.P. (1994) Perceptions of family functioning and cancer. *Psycho-oncology* **3**, 259–269.

Kissane, D.W., Bloch, S., Miach, P., Smith, G.C., Seddon, A. and Keks, N. (1997) Cognitive-existential group therapy for patients with primary breast cancer: techniques and themes. *Psycho-oncology* **6**, 25–34.

Kleinman, A., Eisenberg, L. and Good, B. (1978) Culture, illness and cure. *Ann. Int. Med.* **88**, 251–259.

Koocher, G.P. and O'Malley, J.E. (eds) (1981) *The Damocles syndrome: psychological consequences of surviving childhood cancer.* New York: McGraw-Hill.

Krupnick, J.L., Rowland, J.H., Goldberg, R.L. and Daniel, U.V. (1993) Professionally led support groups for cancer patients: an intervention in search of a model. *Int. J. Psychiatr. Med.* **23**, 275–294.

Kubler-Ross, E. (1969). *On death and dying.* New York: Macmillan.

Lansdown, R. and Goldman, A. (1988) The psychological care of children with malignant disease. *J. Child Psychol. Psychiatr.* **29**, 555–567.

Lansdown, R. and Goldman, A. (1991) Children with cancer. In: M. Watson (ed.), *Cancer patient care: psychosocial treatment methods.* Cambridge: BPS Books and Cambridge University Press, pp. 298–314.

Lazare, A. (1987) Shame and humiliation in the medical encounter. *Arch. Int. Med.* **47**, 1653–1658.

Lesko, L.M. (1993a) Psychiatric aspects of bone marrow transplantation. Part I: special issues during pre-transplant assessment and hospitalization. *Psycho-oncology* **2**, 161–183.

Lesko, L.M. (1993b) Psychiatric aspects of bone marrow transplantation. Part II: life beyond transplant. *Psycho-oncology* **2**, 185–193

Lewis, D.A. and Smith, R.E. (1983) Steroid-induced psychiatric syndromes: a report of 14 cases and a review of the literature. *J. Affect. Dis.* **5**, 319–332.

Lichter, I. (1987) *Communication in cancer care.* Edinburgh: Churchill Livingstone.

Lodge, D. (1991) *Paradise news.* London: Penguin Books.

Loge, J.H., Kaasa, S., Ekeberg, O., Falkum, E. and Hytten, K. (1996) Attitudes toward informing the cancer patient – a survey of Norwegian physicians. *Eur. J. Cancer* **32A**, 1344–1348.

Luborsky, L. (1984) *Principles of psychoanalytic psychotherapy: a manual for supportive-expressive treatment.* New York: Basic Books.

MacNamara, M. (1974) Talking with patients: some problems met by medical students. *Br. J. Med. Educ.* **8**, 17–23.

Maguire, P. (1975) The psychological and social consequences of breast cancer. *Nurs. Mirror* 3 April, 54–57.

Maguire, P. (1980) The repercussions of mastectomy on the family. *Int. J. Family Psychiatr.* **1**, 485–503.

Maguire, P. (1985) Towards more effective psychological intervention in patients with cancer. *Cancer Care* **2**, 12–15.

Maguire, P and Faulkner, A. (1988a) How to do it. Improve the counselling skills of doctors and nurses in cancer care. *Br. Med. J.* **297**, 847–849.

Maguire, P. and Faulkner, A. (1988b). Communicate with cancer patients: 1. Handling bad news and difficult questions. *Br. Med. J.* **297**, 907–909.

Maguire, P. and Faulkner, A. (1988c) Communicate with cancer patients: 2. Handling uncertainty, collusion and denial. *Br. Med. J.* **297**, 972–974.

Maguire, P., Tait, A., Brooke, M., Thomas, C. and Sellwood, R. (1980) Effect of counselling on the psychiatric morbidity association with mastectomy. *Br. Med. J.* **281**, 1454–1456.

Malan, D.H. (1976) *The frontier of brief psychotherapy.* New York: Plenum.

Mann, J. (1973) *Time-limited psychotherapy.* Cambridge: Harvard University Press.

Marks, D.l., Crilley, P., Nezu, C.M. and Nezu, A.M. (1996) Sexual dysfunction prior to high-dose chemotherapy and bone marrow transplantation. *Bone Marrow Transpl.* **17**, 595–599.

McCorkle, R., Yost, L.S., Jepson, C., Malone, D., Baird, S. and Lusk, E. (1993) A cancer experience: relationship of patient psychosocial response to caregiver burden over time. *Psycho-oncology* **2**, 21–32.

McIntosh, J. (1978) The routine management of uncertainty in communication with cancer patients. In: A. Davis (ed.), *Relationships between doctors and patients.* Westmead: Teakfield, pp. 106–131.

McNair, D.M., Lorr, M. and Droppleman, L.F. (1971) *Manual for the profile of mood states.* San Francisco: Educational and Industrial Testing Service.

Meichenbaum, D. (1977) *Cognitive behaviour modification: an integrative approach.* New York: Plenum Press.

Meredith, C., Symonds, P., Webster, L., Lamont, D., Pyper, E., Gillis, C.R. and Fallowfield, L. (1996) Information needs of cancer patients in west Scotland: cross sectional survey of patients' views. *Br. Med. J.* **313**, 724–726.

Messer, S.B. and Warren, C.S. (1995) *Models of brief psychodynamic psychotherapy: A comprehensive approach.* New York: Guilford.

Milton, G.W. (1973) Thoughts in mind of a person with cancer. *Br. Med. J.* 17 October, 221–223.

Mitchell, D.M. and Collins, J.V. (1984) Do corticosteroids really alter mood? *Postgrad. Med. J.* **60**, 467–470.

Molleman, E., Krabbendam, P.J., Annyas, A.A., Koops, H.S., Sleijfer, D.T. and Vermey, A. (1984) The significance of the doctor–patient relationship in coping with cancer. *Soc. Sci. Med.* **18**, 475–480.

Moorey, S. and Greer, S. (1989) *Psychological therapy for patients with cancer: a new approach.* Oxford: Heinemann Medical Books.

Moorey, S., Greer, S., Watson, M., Baruch, J.D.R., Robertson, B.M., Mason, A., Rowden, L., Tunmore, R., Law, M. and Bliss, J.M. (1994) Adjuvant psychological therapy for patients with cancer: one year follow-up of a randomised controlled trial. *Psycho-oncology* **3**, 39–46.

Morrison, B. (1993) *And when did you last see your father?* London: Granta [Penguin].

Morrow, G.R., Hoagland, A.C. and Carpenter, P.J. (1983) Improving physician–patient communications in cancer treatment. *J. Psychosoc. Oncol.* **1**, 93–101.

Mount, B.M. (1986) Dealing with our losses. *J. Clin. Oncol.* **4**, 1127–1134.

Moynihan, C. (1987) Testicular cancer: the psychosocial problems of patients and their relatives. *Cancer Surv.* **6**, 477–510.

Muzzin, L.J., Anderson, N.J., Figeredo, A.T. and Gudelis, S.O. (1994) The experience of cancer. *Soc. Sci. Med.* **38**, 1201–1208.

Mystakidou, K., Liossi, C., Vlachos, L. and Papadimitriou, J. (1996) Disclosure of diagnostic information to cancer patients in Greece. *Palliative Med.* **10**, 195–200.

Nelson, E., Sloper, P., Charlton, A. and While, D. (1994) Children who have a parent with cancer: a pilot study. *J. Cancer Educ.* **9**, 30–36.

Nerenz, D.R., Leventhal, H. and Love, R.R. (1982) Factors contributing to emotional distress during cancer chemotherapy. *Cancer* **50**, 1020–1027.

Northouse, L.L. (1988) Family issues in cancer care. *Adv. Psychosom. Med.* **18**, 82–101.

Northouse, L.L. (1995) The impact of cancer in women on the family. *Cancer Pract.* **3**, 134–142.

Northouse, L.L., Laten, D. and Reddy, P. (1995) Adjustment of women and their husbands to recurrent breast cancer. *Res. Nurs. Health* **18**, 515–524.

O'Connor, A.P., Wicker, C.A. and Germino, B.B. (1990) Understanding the cancer patient's search for meaning. *Cancer Nurs.* **13**, 167–175.

Orbach, C.E., Bard, M. and Sutherland, A.M. (1957) Fears and defensive adaptations to the loss of anal sphincter control. *Psychoanalytic Rev.* **44**, 121–175.

Osler, W. (1906) *Science and immortality.* London: Constable.

Osler, W. (1910) The Lumleian lectures on angina pectoris. *Lancet* **i**, 696–700, 839–844, 974–977.

Ostroff, J.S. and Lesko, L.M. (1991) Psychosexual adjustment and fertility issues. In: M.B. Whedon, (ed.), *Bone marrow transplantation: principles, practice and nursing insights.* Boston: Jones and Bartlett.

Papper, S. (1985) Care of patients with incurable, chronic neoplasm: one patient's perspective. *Am. J. Med.* **78,** 271–276.

Parkes, C.M. (1982) Loss and change: terminal care, bereavement and amputation. In: F. Creedand J. Pfeffer (eds), *Medicine and psychiatry: a practical approach.* London: Pitman, pp. 141–158.

Parkes, C.M. (1996) Bereavement. In: T. Kendrick, A. Tylee and P. Freeling (eds), *The prevention of mental illness in primary care.* Cambridge: Cambridge University Press, pp. 74–87.

Parle, M., Jones, B. and Maguire, P. (1994) Coping with multiple demands of cancer: patients' appraisal patterns, coping responses and mental health [Abstract]. *Psycho-oncology* **3,** 149.

Patel, S. (1996) Preventing mental illness amongst people of ethnic minorities. In: T. Kendrick, A. Tylee and P. Freeling (eds), *The prevention of mental illness in primary care.* Cambridge: Cambridge University Press, pp. 88–112.

Peck, M.S. (1978) *The road less travelled.* New York: Simon & Schuster.

Peteet, J.R. (1985) Religious issues presented by cancer patients seen in psychiatric consultation. *J. Psychosoc. Oncol.* **3,** 53–66.

Peteet, J. and Greenberg, B. (1995) Marital crises in oncology patients: an approach to initial intervention by primary clinicians. *Gen. Hosp. Psychiatr.* **17,** 201–217.

Phillips, L. and Osborne, J. (1989) Cancer patients' experiences of forgiveness therapy. *Can. J. Couns.* **23,** 236–251.

Pistrang, N. and Barker, C. (1995) The partner relationship in psychological response to breast cancer. *Soc. Sci. Med.* **40,** 789–797.

Pronzato, P., Bertelli, G., Losardo, P. and Landucci, M. (1994) What do advanced cancer patients know of their disease? A report from Italy. *Support. Care Cancer* **2,** 242–244.

Quill, T.E. (1995) 'You promised me I wouldn't die like this!' A bad death as a medical emergency. *Arch. Int. Med.* **155,** 1250–1254.

Rait, D. and Lederberg, M. (1989) The family of the cancer patient. In: J.C. Holland and J. Rowland (eds.), *Handbook of Psycho-oncology.* New York: Oxford University Press.

Ream, E. and Richardson, A. (1996) The role of information in patients' adaptation to chemotherapy and radiotherapy: a review of the literature. *Eur. J. Cancer Care* **5,** 132–138.

Reiker, P., Edbril, S. and Garnick, M. (1985) Curative testis cancer therapy: psychosocial sequelae. *J. Clin. Oncol.* **3,** 1117–1126.

Rittenberg, C.N. (1996) Helping children cope when a family member has cancer. *Support. Care Cancer* **4,** 196–199.

Robson, M.H., France, R. and Bland, M. (1984). Clinical psychologist in primary care: controlled clinical and economic evaluation. *Br. Med. J.* **288**, 1805–1808.

Rodrigue, J.R. and Park, T.L. (1996) General and illness-specific adjustment to cancer: relationship to marital status and marital quality. *J. Psychosom. Res.* **40**, 29–36.

Rogers, C. (1951) *Client-centered therapy.* Boston: Houghton Mifflin.

Rogers, C.R. (1957) The necessary and sufficient conditions of therapeutic personality change. *J. Consult. Psychol.* **21**, 95–103.

Schain, W.S. (1981) Self-esteem, sexuality, and cancer management. In: J.G. Goldberg (ed.), *Psychotherapeutic treatment of cancer patients,* New York: Free Press, pp. 316–336.

Schain, W.S. (1988) The sexual and intimate consequences of breast cancer treatment. *CA A Cancer J. for Clinicians* **38**, 154–161.

Schain, W.S. (1990) Physician–patient communication about breast cancer: a challenge for the 1990s. *Surg. Clinics N. America* **70**, 917–936.

Schlesinger, H.J., Mumford, E. and Glass, G.V. (1983) Mental health treatment and medical care utilization in a fee-for-service system: outpatient mental health treatment following the onset of chronic disease. *Am. J. Pub. Health* **73**, 422–429.

Schover, L.R. (1986) Sex and the cancer patient. In: B.A. Stoll and A.D. Weisman (eds), *Coping with cancer stress.* Dordrecht: Martinus Nijhoff, pp. 71–80.

Schover, L.R. and Fife, M. (1985) Sexual counseling of patients undergoing radical surgery for pelvic or genital cancer. *J. Psychosoc. Oncol.* **3**, 21–41.

Schulz, K.H., Schulz, H., Schultz, O. and von Kerekjarto, M. (1996) Family structure and psychosocial stress in families of cancer patients. In: L. Baider, C.L. Cooper and A.K. De-Nour (eds), *Cancer and the family,* Chichester: Wiley, pp. 225–255.

Senescu, R.A. (1963) The development of emotional complications in the patient with cancer. *J. Chronic Dis.* **16**, 813–832.

Shields, P. (1984) Communication: a supportive bridge between cancer patient, family, and healthcare staff. *Nurs. Forum* **21**, 31–36.

Shipes, E. and Lehr, S. (1982) Sexuality and the male cancer patient. *Cancer Nurs.* **4**, 375–381.

Siegel, K., Karus, D. and Raveis, V.H. (1996a) Adjustment of children facing the death of a parent due to cancer. *J. Am. Acad. Child Adol. Psychiatr.* **35**, 442–450.

Siegel, K., Karus, D. and Raveis, V.H. (1996b) Pattern of communication with children when a parent has cancer. In: L. Baider, C.L. Cooper and A.K. De-Nour (eds), *Cancer and the family,* Chichester: Wiley, pp. 109–128.

Siegel, K., Karus, D.G., Raveis, V.H., Christ, G.H. and Mesagno, F.P. (1996) Depressive distress among the spouses of terminally ill cancer patients. *Cancer Pract.* **4**, 25–30.

Skipper, J.K. (1965) Communication and the hospitalized patient. In: J.K. Skipper Jr and R.C. Leonard (eds), *Social interaction and patient care*, Philadelphia: J.B. Lippincott, pp. 61–82.

Slevin, M.L. (1987) Talking about cancer: how much is too much? *Br. J. Hosp. Med.* 38 , **56**, 58–59.

Souhami, R.L. (1978) Teaching what to say about cancer. *Lancet* **ii**, 935–936.

Spiegel, D. (1985) Psychosocial intervention with cancer patients. *J. Psychosoc. Oncol.* **3**, 83–95.

Spiegel, D. (1992) Effects of psychosocial support on patients with metastatic breast cancer. *J. Psychosoc. Oncol.* **10**, 113–120.

Spiegel, D. and Yalom, I. (1978) A support group for dying patients. *Int. J. Group Psychother.* **28**, 233–245.

Sprangers, M.A.G., teVelde, A., Aaronson, N.K. and Taal, B.G. (1993) Quality of life following surgery for colorectal cancer: a literature review. *Psycho-oncology* **2**, 247–259.

Stolbach, L. and Lorman, C. (1994) Further comments on counselling people with cancer: pursuing the perfect paradigm. *Advances* **10**, 57–58.

Strain, J.J. (1978) Psychological reactions to acute medical illness and critical care. *Crit. Care Med.* **6**, 39–44.

Streltzer, J. and Leigh, H. (1978) Psychological preparation for surgery: the usefulness of a preoperative psychotherapeutic interview. *Hawaii Med. J.* **37**, 139–142.

Strupp, H.H. and Binder, J.L. (1984) *Psychotherapy in a new key: a guide to time-limited dynamic psychotherapy.* New York: Basic Books.

Tan, T.K., Teo, F.C., Wong, K. and Lim, H.L. (1993) Cancer: to tell or not to tell? *Singapore Med. J.* **34**, 202–203.

Tarrier, N. and Maguire, P. (1984) Treatment of psychological distress following mastectomy: an initial report. *Behav. Res. Ther.* **22**, 81–84.

Taylor, E.J., Baird, S.B., Malone, D. and McCorkle, R. (1993) Factors associated with anger in cancer patients and their caregivers. *Cancer Pract.* **1**, 101–109.

Thomsen, O.O., Wulff, H.R., Martin, A. and Singer, P.A. (1993) What do gastroenterologists in Europe tell cancer patients? *Lancet* **341**, 473–476.

Trijsberg, R., van Knippenberg, F. and Rijpma, S. (1992) Effects of psychological treatment on cancer patients: a critical review. *Psychosom. Med.* **54**, 489–517.

Trillin, A.S. (1981) Of dragons and garden peas: a cancer patient talks to doctors. *New Eng. J. Med.* **304**, 699–701.

Turk, D.C. and Fernandez, E. (1991) Pain: a cognitive–behavioural perspective. In: M. Watson (ed.), *Cancer patient care: psychosocial treatment methods.* Cambridge: BPS Books and Cambridge University Press, pp. 14–44.

Vachon, M.L.S. (1985) Psychotherapy and the person with cancer: an analysis of one nurse's experience. *Oncol. Nurs. Forum* **12**, 33–40.

Vachon, M.L.S. (1987) Unresolved grief in persons with cancer referred for psychotherapy. *Psychiatr. Clin. N. America* **10**, 467–486.

van Veldhuisen, A.M. and Last, B.F. (1991) *Children with cancer: communication and emotions.* Amsterdam: Swets and Zeitlinger.

Viederman, M. and Perry, S.W. (1980) Use of a psychodynamic life narrative in the treatment of depression in the physically ill. *Gen. Hosp. Psychiatr.* 3, 177–185.

Viney, L. (1983) *Images of illness.* Krieger.

Vugia, H. (1991) Support groups in oncology: building hope through the human bond. *J. Psychosoc. Oncol.* **9**, 89–107.

Watson, M. (1984) The effectiveness of specialist nurses as oncology counsellors. In Watson, M. and Greer, S. (eds), *Psychosocial issues in malignant disease.* Oxford: Pergamon.

Watson, M., Greer, S., Blake, S. and Shrapnell, K. (1984) Reaction to a diagnosis of breast cancer: relationship between denial, delay and rates of psychological morbidity. *Cancer* **53**, 2008–2012.

Watson, M., Greer, S., Rowden, L., Gorman, C., Robertson, B., Bliss, J.M. and Tunmore, R. (1991) Relationships between emotional control, adjustment to cancer and depression and anxiety in breast cancer patients. *Psychol. Med.* **21**, 51–57.

Watson, M., McCarron, J. and Law, M. (1992) Anticipatory nausea and emesis and psychological morbidity: assessment of prevalence among outpatients on mild to moderate chemotherapy regimens. *Br. J. Cancer* **66**, 862–866.

Watson, M., Law, M., dos Santos, M., Greer, S., Baruch, J. and Bliss, J. (1994) The Mini-MAC: further development of the Mental Adjustment to Cancer Scale. *J. Psychosoc. Oncol.* **12**, 33–46.

Watson, M., Fenlon, D. and McVey, G. (1996) A support group for breast cancer patients: development of a cognitive–behavioural approach. *Behav. Cogn. Psychother.* **24**, 73–81.

Watts, E.J. (1993) Communicating with children and teenagers with cancer – difficult for the doctor but worse for the patient. *Psychooncology* **2**, 285–287.

Weihs, K. and Reiss, D. (1996) Family reorganization in response to cancer: a developmental perspective. In: L. Baider, C.L. Cooper and A.K. De-Nour (eds), *Cancer and the family*, Chichester, Wiley, pp. 3–29.

Weil, M., Smith, M. and Khayat, D. (1994) Truth-telling to cancer patients in the Western European context. *Psycho-oncology* 3, 21–26.

Weisman, A.D. (1979a) *Coping with cancer*. New York: McGraw-Hill.

Weisman, A.D. (1979b) A model for psychosocial phasing in cancer. *Gen. Hosp. Psychiatr.* 1, 187–195.

Weisman, A.D. and Worden, J.W. (1976–7) The existential plight in cancer: significance of the first 100 days. *Int. J. Psychiatr. Med.* 7, 1–15.

Wellisch, D.K., Gritz, E.R., Schain, W., Wang, H.J. and Siau, J. (1992) Psychological functioning of daughters of breast cancer patients. Part II: characterizing the distressed daughter of the breast cancer patient. *Psychosomatics* 33, 171–179.

Wellisch, D.K., Hoffman, A. and Gritz, E. (1996) Psychological concerns and care of daughters of breast cancer patients. In: L. Baider, C.L. Cooper and A.K. De-Nour (eds), *Cancer and the family*, Chichester: Wiley, pp. 289–304.

Winnicott, D.W. (1965) *The maturational processes and the facilitating environment.* New York: International Universities Press.

Wool, M.S. and Goldberg, R.J. (1986) Assessment of denial in cancer patients: implications forintervention. *J. Psychosoc. Oncol.* 4, 1–14.

Worden, J.W. (1983) *Grief counselling and grief therapy.* London: Tavistock.

Worden, J.W. and Weisman, A.D. (1980) Do cancer patients really want counselling? *Gen. Hosp. Psychiat.* 2, 100–103.

Zigmond, A.S. and Snaith, R.P. (1983) The Hospital Anxiety and Depression Scale. *Acta Psychiatr. Scand.* 67, 361–370.

Zilbergeld, B. (1979) Sex and serious illness. In: C.A. Garfield (ed.) *Stress and survival: the emotional realities of life-threatening illness.* St Louis: Mosby, pp. 236–242.

Index

Activity scheduling 153
AIDS 61
Androgen deficiency 68
Anger 40–2, 144
Anti-depressants 159
Adjustment 34
Adjustment disorder 26
Anticipatory nausea and
    vomiting 24
Anxiety 27
  measures 173
Anxious preoccupation 35

BACUP 23, 126
Behavioural techniques 152–4
Bereavement 111–12
Body image 58
Bone marrow transplant 24
Booklets 23
Breaking bad news 75–8
  aligning 80
  enabling 85
  reflective technique 85
  the warning shot 79
  window of opportunity 84

Cancer treatments 15, 23
  chemotherapy 23

radiotherapy 23
surgery 18
Catheters 58
Children 50
  adolescent 51
  preadolescent 50
  withholding information 51
Chronic sorrow 31
Clergy 97
Client-centred therapy 126, 149
  general principles 126
  model 126
  reflecting feelings 132, 148
  unconditional positive regard
    137
Closure 88
Cognitive avoidance 35
Cognitive–behavioural therapy
    150–52
  model 150
Cognitive techniques 155–9
Colostomy 31, 58, 65
Communication 69
  disclosing the diagnosis
    69–75
  disengagement 87
  distancing techniques 85–7,
    136
  ethical principle 75

Communication (*cont.*)
  euphemisms 70
  resistance to listening 134
  the terminally ill 85–6,
    102–10
Confidentiality 175
Conspiracy of silence 47–8
Control 8, 122, 143
Coping 34
  styles 34–6, 148
Counselling contract 176
Countertransference 118
Couples 55–6
  estranged 56
  hostile-dependent 55
  immature 55

Damocles
  sword of 97
  syndrome 16
Death and dying 102–10, 135
  information giving 103
  staff coping 106 (Table)
  stages 102
Denial 35–8, 74
Dependency 143
Depression 32
  measures 173
  postoperative 20
Disease stage 14

Eastern medicine 52
Economic measures 174
Ego strength 22
Empathic listening 138
Empathy 4, 137
Ethical consultant 32
Ethnic groups 52
Existential 11, 30
  crisis 96
  issues 30
  plight 11

Families 43
  ambivalent 48
  at risk 48
  disengaged 49
  disorganized 48
  dynamics 54
  enmeshed 49
  hostile 49
  of the terminally ill 105
  supportive 48
Fatalism 35
Fighting spirit 35

General Health Questionnaire
  174
Giving up-given up complex
  65, 95
Graft-versus-host disease 25
Grief 95
  anticipatory 96, 107
  reactions 95–6, 108–9
  unresolved 95
Groups 160
  audit 169
  implementation 164
  nondirective 161–2
  planning 163
  professionally-led 160
  psychoeducational 160–61
  support 160

Haematological malignancies 24
Helplessness 30, 35
Homosexual men 65
Hormonal Therapies 24
Hospital Anxiety and Depression
  Scale 174
Hospital chaplain 32

Information-giving 89
Informed consent 91
Interpersonal issues 142–6

Intimacy 143
Isolation 25, 46

Life events 94
Loss 116
Lumpectomy 67

Malan's model 118
Mastectomy 67
Metaphors 146
Minimizing 39

Negative automatic thoughts
   158
Noncompliance 6, 32, 39

Occupational stress 110
Oestrogen deficiency 68

Partners 44–5
   as co-therapist 154
Personality Type 8 (Table)
PLISSIT model 62
Profile of Mood States 174
Psychodynamic 113–25
   formulation 123, 125
   life narrative 113–17
   model 113
   therapists 117
   therapy 113
Psychological problems 28
   increased risk 28–9
   partners 46
   themes 29
Psychosexual Issues 56, 59
   (Table), 144
   colorectal cancer 63
   colostomy 62

ileal conduit 64
   mastectomy 66–7
Psychotherapy
   and internal object
      relationships 121
   contract model 121
   dynamic focus 121
   supportive-expressive 120
   time-limited 120

Regression 5, 110
Rejection 145

Self-disclosure 144
Separation 145
Service evaluation 172–3
Sexual dysfunction 56
   assessment of 56–7
   impotence 64, 65
Sexual health 60
Sexual history 61
Significant other 44
Social support 29
   system 44
Spiritual issues 97
Steroids 25
Stigma 45
Stoic acceptance 35
Suicide 28
Summarizing 89
Supervision 174

Tamoxifen 25
Terminal illness 99
   and feelings 101
Transference 117
Treatment decisions 91–2
Trust 143

Printed in the United States
117728LV00004B/213/A